50 is the new 20

A step-by-step guide to longevity

January 2022

Table of Contents

Copyright 2

Introduction 3

Chapter 1 - Be an Athlete of Life 7

Chapter2 - The Courage to Fail 13

Chapter 3: Sitting is the New Smoking 18

Chapter 4: Watch How Others Live the Last Years of Life 23

Chapter 5: Change Now 27

Chapter 6: Inflammation, Sleep, Stress 34

Chapter 7: Metabolic Dysfunction 45

Chapter 8: Lift Weights 59

Chapter 9: Limit Meds 64

Chapter 10: Stretch 69

Chapter 11: Go Outside 73

Chapter 12: Hydration 76

Chapter 13: Alcohol 81

Chapter 14: Added Sugar 84

Chapter 15: BPAs, PFAs, Plastics and Other Forever Chemicals 91

Chapter 16: A Typical Day 101

Chapter 17: Bio-Hacks 104

Conclusion 106

About The Author 107

Copyright

Copyright © January 2022 by Mathew Barry

All rights reserved. No part of this publication may be reproduced, distributed, or transmitted in any form or by any means, including photocopying, recording, or other electronic or mechanical methods, without the prior written permission of the author, except in the case of brief quotations embodied in critical reviews and certain other noncommercial uses permitted by copyright law.

For permission requests, email the author at: doctormbarry@gmail.com

This work is intended to be educational. As such, quotations and data from other sources are used under the Fair Use Doctrine of United States Copyright Law. Notation and full credit is given for the originator of each quotation or data source.

Edit and formatting by WritingAllsorts

First edition published January 2022

ISBN-13: (Softcover) 9798402482104

Introduction

For more than two decades I have dedicated a vast portion of my life to searching for ways to improve the health, performance, and the well-being of my patients, clients, and myself. My professional journey began as a Certified Strength and Conditioning Specialist working with athletes ranging from high school to the Olympic and professional ranks. This led me to further my education by pursuing a graduate and post graduate degree, eventually becoming a Doctor of Physical Therapy.

During this time, I studied and implemented treatments gleaned from peer-reviewed studies, while also completing research of my own. For me, the next logical step was to share the knowledge that I gained with everyone who would listen. I became an adjunct professor for the Physical Therapist Assistant program at Sacramento City College, teaching students in subjects ranging from neurological disorders to pathopysiology.

Fast forward a few years. In my quest to reach a much wider audience, I have decided to share the things I have learned by writing this book.

My goal with this book is to pass on the information that I have gained, allowing me to offer you some insights and strategies to improve your health. You're at least a little bit interested in learning ways to better your fitness, or you wouldn't have opened this book. I've realized as I've gotten older, that maintaining a healthy lifestyle can be difficult and I'm sure a lot of you feel the same way. Unfortunately, our bodies don't always work like they did when we were in our twenties. Like the title states, what I hope to show is that by implementing certain habits into our lives, we can get back to that level of function. I'll do my best to demonstrate this by using the most current data through peer-reviewed studies so as to avoid any confusion, or debate. I include anecdotes, evidence found on various popular websites as well as personal experience to help illustrate certain points.

As we all know, things change in science. What is known today, can change in the future as more studies are completed. However, based on the latest knowledge, we can ascertain ways to maximize one's *healthspan* (a theme that will be revisited throughout this book) to be as fit and as functional for as long as possible.

I'll try to keep the tone light, as trudging through study after study can be tedious and really boring. In no way am I trying to downplay certain situations, or circumstances that some of you may be in, through no fault of your own. I'll also do my best to be as compassionate as possible since one never knows what their health may be like in the future. A lot of what I state is common sense, but it never hurts to hear it again in terms that may be a bit easier to understand.

I recognize that the strategies I present may not work best for everyone, and I've found that humility can open my eyes to other options that I may have overlooked or ignored altogether. I try to practice this throughout the book, and I hope it shows. I can appreciate that others may have found methods that work for them and their clients or may be familiar with a study or a technique that I'm not familiar with. To them I say keep up the good work.

I understand that there are other opinions and strategies being used by some. What is presented, in my professional experience, is what I have found produces the best results for my patients and clients.

Please forgive me if it seems that the book is slanted toward an American point of view. I do live in America, therefore most of my perspectives are that of an American. This book, however, is for anyone and everyone, no matter what country you live in. Many of my quotes and citations are from authors from all over the world, and I do my best to include view points from all countries.

I have purposefully kept this book short and to the point and I have tried my best to not present the information in a condescending fashion. There are many other books and studies, which I will cite throughout, that go way deeper in detail on the various topics I've presented. I encourage you to further investigate them. My goal is to consolidate and summarize the things that I feel are most important and present them in ways that are actionable. This will allow you to understand and implement the forthcoming findings as soon as possible into your daily lives in a way that's right for you.

It's never too late to start getting healthier and by reading this you've already taken a step in the right direction.

Please keep in mind, I am in no way suggesting these ideas form a patient-doctor/clinician relationship, and you should always consult with your physician and/or healthcare professional before starting any health improvement program.

Chapter 1 - Be an Athlete of Life

We've all felt that sinking feeling of thinking we could do something, only to find out unceremoniously that we no longer can. For instance, you go to a home improvement store to pick up a few things for a project. You bend down to pick up the 50lb bag of concrete that you need and, BOOM! there goes your back. Or what about bending down to pick up your grandkid, only to realize that she's gotten too heavy to do so (i.e. Your muscles have gotten too weak to do so). Now, you're probably standing there alarmed, wondering, *how did this happen?*

Obviously, as we age, we go through a few things physically that may necessitate modifications, but age should NOT stop us from doing the everyday things we need to do (aka activities of daily living, or ADLs for short).

One of my main drivers of continuing a healthy lifestyle is so I can do whatever activity I want, without being incredibly sore, or without getting injured. If you can't pick up your grandkid in your fifties or make it up a flight of stairs in your teens or twenties without being out of breath, that's a problem.

My father-in-law once lamented that he regrets, due to injury, no longer being able to go on walks with my nephew. The sadness in his voice was palpable. Yes, he's in his early seventies, but not even being able to walk a few hundred feet when your grandson is pleading with you has got to be heart-breaking.

To steal a line I heard from longevity specialist and podcaster Dr. Peter Attia, "Be an athlete of life." This doesn't mean the world should expect you to match your max bench press, or your 40-yard-dash time from when you were twenty-five (although you absolutely can if you play your cards right). It does mean that you definitely should be able to pick up a 50lb bag of cement, or your grandkid, without being laid-up for a week. Some simple training and activity techniques, along with consistency, can keep you strong enough to complete ADLs with no repercussions.

Strengthening your muscles is a must to reduce the risk of muscle atrophy and possibly *sarcopenia* (severe muscle wasting). Unfortunately, decreased muscle mass happens to us all, typically starting at age thirty (please see bio-hacks section for tips to increase testosterone and human growth hormone, aka HGH, the precursor to growth and maintenance). This can lead to all kinds of issues, like falls, fractures, and being unable to pick up light objects.

Before I go any further, let me explain the term "bio-hack". This term was coined recently by those of us interested in finding ways to improve our bodies function through science and technology. Think of it as ways to get around the perceived limits that have been placed on our bodies by finding new and innovative strategies to re-charge our biological abilities. This can be taken to the extreme, as some people have done things like injecting themselves with chemicals or small instruments. However, for most of us, it is implementing new and/or old and forgotten tactics into our daily habits to rediscover the health and vitality we enjoyed when we were younger.

Easy actions like taking daily walks can keep your body strong and your cardiovascular system running smoothly. The benefits of walking, as stated by the Mayo Clinic, are many: bone health improves, as well as balance. The risk of heart attack, stroke, and type 2 diabetes plummets as can the symptoms of depression.[1] These improvements can allow you to do more functional activities, or ADLs, for a longer time, as well as help maintain your *optimal* level of health.

An easy muscle maintenance program can be done in surprisingly simple ways. Have stairs? Use the bottom step and do ten step-ups per leg for a few sets. No steps; go outside and step up and down the curb, or a park bench for more of a challenge. Lay on your back with your knees bent and pick your hips up off the floor for twenty repetitions (these are called bridges, my absolute favorite exercise of all time). Or get on the ground and do a few pushups.

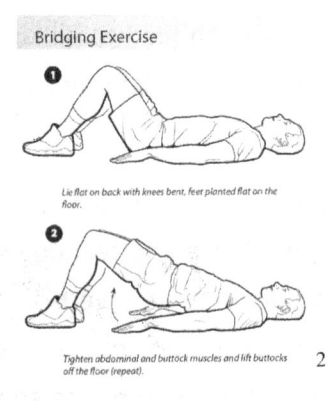

Bridging Exercise

❶

Lie flat on back with knees bent, feet planted flat on the floor.

❷

Tighten abdominal and buttock muscles and lift buttocks off the floor (repeat).

2

---

[1] https://www.mayoclinic.org/healthy-lifestyle/fitness/in-depth/walking/art-20046261

Find a good physical therapist, certified strength and conditioning specialist (CSCS), or an educated personal trainer to get you set up on a proper program. Just be sure your goals are clear, achievable, and realistic so that you don't get discouraged. Don't just say, "I want to be able to run the forty-yard-dash like I did at twenty-five," knowing full well you've had a few knee surgeries and haven't run in ten years. You'll quit faster than you ran the forty-yard-dash when you were twenty-five.

Start by committing to exercise two or three days/week for one month. This can be as easy as going on a 30-minute walk three times per week. Once that one's knocked down, set up the next goal:

'I'll be able to complete twenty-five pushups non-stop within the next four weeks.' Knock it down, set up the next.

A couple of quotes I like to live by:

The first was from former Olympian and heavyweight boxing champion Evander Holyfield. He was always one of my role-models for a healthy body as he always remained in great shape throughout his career. He was once asked his secret, which lead to this simple response:

"It's easier to stay in shape than to get into shape."

---

[2] http://physioprofessionals.com.au/wp-content/uploads/2015/10/Bridging-Exercise.jpg?x54680

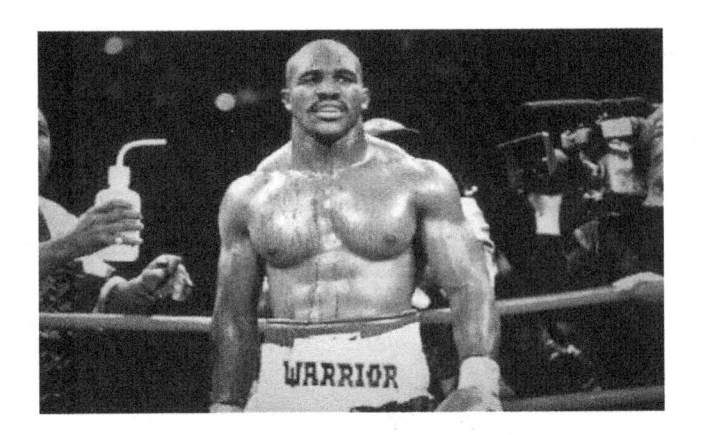

This resonated with me, and from the time I was eighteen, I did my best to never get out of shape. I consistently lifted weights and did my best to eat healthy foods and live a healthy lifestyle. In no way am I comparing myself to a professional athlete. Most of us will never achieve that level, and most of us likely have much different goals than to look like Mr. Holyfield. However, that simple quote helped motivate me to stay consistent.

Another great quote is from country music artist Toby Keith: "Don't let the old man in."

Preach! Being 'fifty' is just a number. In no way, shape, or form do I *think* I'm fifty. It never really crosses my mind, nor does the expectations of what a fifty-year-old should look and act like. Of course, every now and then I get reminded that I'm no spring chicken, however, I never dwell on that. I don't let the old man in! When I hang out with people my age, there are times I just have to excuse myself, as some of them dwell on how everything hurts, or how they used to be able to do this or that. They sound as if they've given up already. The 'old man' has not only gotten in, he's comfortably kicked back on his recliner, watching the TV with a beer in his hand.

I'm sure this isn't the first time you've read or heard this. The difference is, you need to understand that time and youth are no longer on your side. This may be revealed to you when you need to pick something up that used to be easy, yet now it is more difficult than you remember. Next thing you know you're calling for help and your ego is bruised. And that, ladies and gentlemen, is something I'm hoping to help you avoid.

Getting healthier may be tough, but please believe that not being healthy can be tougher. Find what motivates you to live a healthier life. No need to dwell so much on how you look. Be more concerned with how you feel and how you function. A healthier look will be the by-product of the pursuit of overall health. Make a conscious effort to get more fit so that you can be a good grandparent, teammate, husband/wife, father/mother, or athlete of life.

Chapter2 - The Courage to Fail

When I was forty-six, I moved from Northern California to beautiful San Diego with the full intention of taking up surfing, if not daily, then as much as I possibly could. I have surfed intermittently throughout my life since I was ten, but never consistently. That is to say, I never got beyond the beginner level. Shortly after settling in, I eagerly ran out and bought a second-hand surfboard and paddled out into the Pacific.

Talk about a titanic ego crusher! I learned very quickly, that you do not look cool when you're learning, and learning lasts for a long time. It's both mentally and physically taxing, and at times, dangerous. This is where having *the courage to fail,* to not give up, really gets tested. For weeks I tried my hardest, yet I was out there floundering about like an anguished seal, worried that at any moment I'd become a shark's lunch.

Now fast forward three years. I'm a few years closer to fifty and my ego still gets crushed multiple times per week. However, I can now hold my own surfing fairly well and have progressed beyond what I thought I could, based on my initial few sessions.

Speaking of ego, it makes some people do some really stupid things, sometimes in a good way, other times, not so much. Something most of us have learned through life experience is how to over-ride our egos' chatter.

Taking a quote from former Navy SEAL and current U.S. Congressman Dan Crenshaw:

"A life unchallenged by hardship is a missed opportunity... therefore seek to do something hard." - *Fortitude*[3]

I'm no Navy SEAL, but I have taken Congressman Crenshaw's advice to heart. Most things that are easy don't get you to where you strive to be. Doing hard stuff will embarrass you, make you sore, crush your ego, and maybe get you injured. But it can also make you physically and mentally stronger. It can earn you respect amongst peers, or maybe result in a raise from completing a difficult work task others were afraid to take on. It will generally make you feel like you can do just about anything you put your mind to.

I'm sure you have experienced the feeling of accomplishment when finishing something that was very difficult, whether it was an important project for work, or a weekend project around the house. Opportunity for hardship accepted, and challenge met. No one gets recognition for

---

[3] Fortitude: American Resilience in the Era of Outrage. Dan Crenshaw. Grand Central Publishing. April, 2020

finishing an ice cream cone as it's not hard to do. But the recognition you receive after finishing a triathlon? That is well earned.

With that said, please use common sense when pursuing a new endeavor. As we age, injuries can be a major setback that could hinder us for the rest of our lives. Use the wisdom you've gained through the years to help you figure out ways to master these new objectives, and don't be afraid to fail. You have undoubtedly made plenty of mistakes in the past. Success comes from learning from these mistakes and using that knowledge to propel you toward your goals.

I know this is an obvious statement, but it is so much easier to stay dedicated to a health or workout plan if it's something you like to do, or if it is something you are good at. I know not everyone loves going to the gym to fight for space and equipment. Getting up at 5 am gets old real quick. Running just plain sucks. I get it.

Unfortunately, no one has figured out a way to optimize your overall health without putting in some work. There are scientists that are definitely trying, but until then, nothing beats hard work.

I'm a bit unusual in that I actually like going to the gym and exercising in general. Don't get me wrong, I can sit around and watch eight hours of football with the best of 'em on any given Sunday. But for the most part, I don't like to sit still.

Although, I can still fall into a rut where I do the same easy things over and over for weeks or months before I realize that I'm just going through the motions. It's something easy and I'm good at it. At that point, I re-think my routine and mix it up. If I've been squatting the same weight for weeks, I'll throw on an extra 50 lbs. and watch my legs shake as I struggle to lift it. This is good for both my mental and physical being, not to mention it can bring some humility back to my life.

I've learned as I've gotten older, to not be afraid of bombing. I've found the *courage to fail.*

When I turned forty, I was looking for a new challenge. While I didn't get all emotional, or have a mid-life crisis, I did realize it was time for something different. I tried out for an adult league baseball team.

They say baseball is a game of failure, and boy is that true. If you can be successful at the plate 30 percent of the time, you're a hall-of-famer. Mind you, I hadn't played an organized game of baseball since I was probably thirteen years old. The good news, at forty I was still in pretty good shape so I knew I wouldn't embarrass myself athletically, but I was worried about how I would react to the first curveball thrown at me in twenty-seven years. Taking that first step onto the diamond was intimidating, but doing so not only satisfied the drive and passion that I've always had for competition, it rekindled my love for the game of baseball. I was eventually named captain of that team and continue to play to this day.

As for the surfing? I'm lucky enough to live within walking distance to my local surf break. I surf pretty much every day and still get butterflies before I paddle out. The adrenaline rush of dropping in on a big wave will never get old. It brings me tons of joy as well as a fun way to stay physically fit. Just think if I would've quit after the first few days of soul-crushing wipeouts. I would have never met the numerous people that I now call friends. I would have never been able to tell people about the time a shark swam beneath my board and I (really) nor would I continue to experience the ocean and all of its beauty the way only a surfer can. And yes, I still embarrass myself here and there, but I've learned to not let it bother me.

Find the courage to get out of your comfort zone. You may have always wanted to try Jiu-Jitsu, but were too afraid you would get your butt kicked so you never started. You may have always loved playing basketball, but thought you were too old so you just stuck to watching it instead.

Bottom line: Finding ways to challenge yourself will likely require you to get out of your comfort zone. Don't be afraid to fail. Use the wisdom and experience you've gained over the years to keep your spirits up and learn from those failures. I've worked to find a few different things that I like to do, that also keep me healthy, physically active and in good shape. Surely you can too.

So, take a breath and walk into that Jiu-Jitsu gym and have some fun. Jump in the pool and learn how to swim so you can complete your first triathlon. Get out of your comfort zone, do something hard and have the courage to fail.

Chapter 3: Sitting is the New Smoking

I think we're all familiar now with the hazards of cigarette smoking. We are aware that inhaling the myriad carcinogens that are packed into that little tube of death can wreak havoc on our bodies, resulting in devastating diseases such as cancers, hypertension, heart attacks, and strokes, to name a few.

Research has shown that a sedentary lifestyle can be as damaging to your health as smoking, as it can lead to issues such as increased weight and obesity. About one in five deaths is caused each year by obesity (likely more during the COVID-19 era), which is nearly as many as smoking [4]

Remember, our bodies are made to move. We have evolved over hundreds of thousands of years living and surviving by hunting, gathering and following migrating herds for food. Some anthropologists will point out that these hunter/gatherers indeed had some down time, and I agree with that. But they didn't sit around on their sofas mindlessly watching TV. They didn't sit at a desk all day hunched over staring at a computer screen. Cavemen didn't sit in their car while commuting an hour to and from work, stressed out gripping the steering wheel while yelling at traffic for decades until they reached retirement age.

---

[4] https://pubmed.ncbi.nlm.nih.gov/23948004/

Others may be quick to point out that they had to deal with dinosaurs and disease.

Understood. But have you ever seen a depiction of an obese caveman? Maybe they existed, but I guarantee they were the first to be eaten by said dinosaur, as they likely couldn't outrun their less rotund counterparts.

I digress. Since dinosaurs are extinct, and we have a pretty good supply of antibiotics, we'll focus on today's issues, thank you. Simply put, the effects of a sedentary lifestyle can be every bit as devastating as puffing on that cigarette.

The good news: smoking is at an all-time low in the United States. However, the same can't be said for inactivity.

According to a recent survey conducted by Stanford University, the U.S. is tenth among countries for physical activity.[5] In contrast, BBC news reports, Uganda is the most physically active.[6] That study suggests this is because Ugandans spend more time walking (to work and otherwise) and have more physically demanding jobs.

---

[5] https://www.forbes.com/sites/niallmccarthy/2017/07/20/the-worlds-most-and-least-active-countries-infographic/?sh=588df0013a26

[6] https://www.bbc.com/news/world-africa-45496654.

Further, according to a study published in the *Journal of American Medicine,* forty percent of Americans are obese.[7] Some other studies that I've read have stated three out of four Americans are overweight, or obese. Don't believe me? Next time you're out in public, just look around. Please do not take this as me 'fat-shaming.' I am just reporting data and what my eyes see.

Inactivity, and moreover obesity, can lead to many of the same issues smoking causes (hypertension, strokes, heart attacks, and cancers).

Think of the disparity of access to food, gyms, education, etc., that we have here in the U.S. compared to a place like Uganda. This is no knock on Uganda, by any means (they obviously make the best out of everything they have available to them). The point is, we may have state-of-the-art gyms, and places to buy food just a few steps away, and some of the highest access to the internet of any country, yet, we are fat and lazy, and it's getting worse. Oh, and Uganda's obesity rate? 2.3% [8]

Additionally, our medical costs for treatment are astronomical. A 2016 study found that the cost of treating obesity was $149 billion![9] Think of what we could do if we cut that in half. Surely, after 2020 and the

---

[7] https://www.usnews.com/news/healthiest-communities/articles/2019-09-19/obesity-in-america-a-guide-to-the-public-health-crisis .
[8] https://pubmed.ncbi.nlm.nih.gov/21416039/

[9] https://www.usnews.com/news/healthiest-communities/articles/2019-09-19/obesity-in-america-a-guide-to-the-public-health-crisis

pandemic restrictions that led to a decrease in activity, that number is even higher.

Perhaps even more disturbing is a recent study by the CDC stating: "Obesity prevalence was 13.4% among 2- to 5-year-olds, 20.3% among 6- to 11-year-olds, and 21.2% among 12- to 19-year-olds."[10] To clarify, one in five kids aged six-nineteen are obese!

So, what can be done about this?

I've listed a few actionable things that I have found make a huge difference, ranging from simple and inexpensive, to relatively expensive.

- Bike or walk to work. Of course, this may not always be possible (especially if you are working from home) but the physical AND mental benefits of not sitting in your car stressed out in traffic can be enormous.
- Try taking phone/conference calls while standing up, or better yet, while walking. I know you may need your computer in front of you to see numbers, graphs, etc., but if you don't, get out of your chair. Also, most phones are able to pull up those graphs and numbers, so put in your earpiece and get going.

---

[10] https://www.cdc.gov/obesity/data/childhood.html

- Take the stairs when able. We all know this and have heard it before, but it's so relevant. You may be muttering "but I work on the thirty-fifth floor..." Okay. How about starting with walking up to the second floor and catching the elevator from there, then progressing higher and higher.
- Get a standing desk. Standing, rather than sitting, incorporates many more muscles and promotes movement and blood flow that doesn't happen while seated (you'll burn more calories standing).
- Can't get a standing desk? Set a recurring timer on your phone for every thirty minutes that reminds you to stand up. While doing so, take a few deep breaths, do a few calf raises, march in place, squat, etc.
- Enroll your kids in a sports program, or at least make them put down the iPad and go outside for thirty minutes or more daily. I know this book is about us and not our kids, but it never hurts to start this lifestyle early.

Start thinking of ways you can start doing something to better yourself and maybe do your part to help get your nation's obesity level down near Uganda's. Your body will thank you.

Chapter 4: Watch How Others Live the Last Years of Life

In my profession, I have the ability to watch how people live the last few years of their lives in different ways. The disparity is amazing to see. I've seen some age gracefully and pass on peacefully and content. Unfortunately, I've seen others who have suffered for days, or even years until their final breath, some through no fault of their own, others due to circumstances that they put themselves in. I know which way I want to go out.

In a lot of cultures, death is a touchy subject. Of course, there are a tremendous number of variables that go in to the dying process. One could step off a curb and get hit by a bus in their twenties, or fall off a ladder and never recover. Please understand that I am not making light of this matter, or being insensitive. We all die. Father time is undefeated. I just want to try to paint a picture here that we have a bit of control over the end of life process and how aging goes.

I've heard many times, people bragging about how when they were kids, they would, "Drink out of the hose and are just fine!" or "Never put on sunscreen" or "Ride bikes all day without a helmet", etc. While I did these things as well, I realize how they can, and may, impact me going forward. Now, I'm not saying that if you drank out of a hose you're doomed. But, I am saying that these things that we did while we were younger, will affect us as we get older. One of the many concussions I received came when I crashed on my bike and bounced my head off the asphalt, sans helmet.

If you made it a habit to drink from a chemically unsafe utensil, be it a hose or a BPA ridden bottle, your body will be affected somehow, someway. It could manifest itself in a decreased level of testosterone at an earlier than expected age. It could also present as cancer. I'm being a bit dramatic, I understand, but just making a point.

Let's pretend at the age of seventy-five you are bed-ridden and in pain with no chance of improvement. At that moment, your lifespan probably isn't something you're interested in increasing. However, if you were able to change those last few years into being functionally independent (having an increased *health span*) I would bet my bottom dollar that you would have.

Some will argue that, "I'm going to die anyway, why not have fun?" Right, but it's the *way you die* that I care about. Don't you want to go out peacefully and with as little pain and discomfort as possible? Of course you do. If you have smoked your entire life, I will bet that more likely than not, the end of your life is going to be rough. Further, the burden you put on your family (or your country) who may have to cover your care, can be tremendous. I've seen families struggle financially, emotionally, and physically trying to care for a loved one who is dying slowly and distressed.

Again, it's not necessarily your lifespan that you should worry about. Instead, focus on your health span. Remember the chapter about being an athlete of life? That goes hand-in-hand with health span. I want to be able to do whatever I want at any age, be it playing with my grandkids, or picking up that bag of cement. The ability to walk on the beach, or take vacations at an increased age is all part of a vigorous health span.

This has changed the way I think about a lot of things. I have made a choice to do better at taking care of myself so as to avoid these pitfalls when my time comes. I do not want to be a burden on my wife and children, so I do my best now to make choices that will help ensure that outcome. I could absolutely still do better, but I do better than most and continually look for ways to improve.

Try tamping down your inner voice that's telling you, "I've been doing this for years; I'm not stopping now."

That attitude can lead to one continuing to drink sugary sodas, or smoking, or microwaving food in plastic containers. Progressing down that road will likely lead to you being stuck on the couch, wheezing your way through life from your fifties until you die. Your lung function will obviously suffer from smoking (among the many other health issues) while your metabolic health will suffer from those sugary drinks leading to excess weight or obesity, which will be exacerbated by your low testosterone from the endocrine system disruption courtesy of the plastics. All the while, you may be watching your peers or older counterparts who made appropriate changes, continue on with an active lifestyle. Think about running around with your grandkids, or keeping up with your own kids, or even progressing athletically in whatever endeavor you enjoy. These activities will be affected by your lifestyle choices. It's up to you which way it goes.

You at least have a mild interest in changing, or you probably wouldn't be reading this book. You can do it. Its' never too late to start. Try choosing one thing that you will change this week/month/year and do it. Find another, and another and make the change.

Chapter 5: Change Now

You have probably told your kids, or someone younger than you, "You'll be my age faster than you think," or something to that regard. I remember in my twenties thinking that a fifty-year-old has one foot in the grave. Well, here I am and it only seems like yesterday I was thinking that.

Let's face it, most of us were pretty stupid in our twenties. If we could go back, I guarantee all of us would tell our younger self to change something that would benefit us now. Some of us would tell our young self to invest 15 percent in a 401(k), or buy a stock called Amazon ASAP! Others would maybe tell that punk son-of-a-gun that all this partying is going to wreak havoc on their older self and, for the love of God, chillout! Still, others might beg the kid to start exercising and eating right.

Well *that* can't happen, but you can still start NOW. You already know this. Starting to invest in a 401(k) is always a good idea at any age, as is starting any type of exercise, or clean eating program. It will reap benefits almost immediately.

If you were like many folks, you may have started an exercise program when COVID-19 hit. Well, one year later, your body was better for it. Unfortunately, it seems most people actually gained weight and did less. According to a WebMD study, fifty-five percent of men gained weight (with more than half of those men gaining 7lbs or more)[11]

This will be a problem both now, and in the future for these people if something isn't done quickly. For example, a 200 lb. man exerts 1.5x his body weight on his knees while walking, and up to three times body weight when going up/down stairs.[12] This results in increased risk for arthritis, which will lead to decreased activity due to pain, which will lead to increased weight, which will lead to increased arthritis. You get the picture.

Further, increased fat mass leads to increased inflammation throughout the body. This is a huge issue that's not being talked about enough. Systemic inflammation can lead to all kinds of health issues, from cancer to Alzheimer's (more on that in the next chapter).

Enough with the doom-and-gloom. The good news is if you start doing something NOW, you can affect all of these risk factors. Start by just going for a walk. Increase your distance and time as you're able. Did you know that one of the best ways to control blood sugar and reduce your diabetes risk is to walk after each meal? Your muscles will burn some of the glucose that's streaming through your body after you eat, resulting in lower blood glucose levels and decreased diabetes risk. More on this as well in upcoming chapters.

---

[11] https://www.webmd.com/lung/news/20200518/webmd-poll-many-report-weight-gain-during-shutdown

[12] https://www.health.harvard.edu/pain/why-weight-matters-when-it-comes-to-joint-pain

Gradually increase your exercises by doing push-ups a few times per day or step up and down a curb. When you're done with this chapter, stand up and down ten times from the chair you may be sitting in. While the stress on your knees initially may be an issue, your body will respond by building muscle and adapting to this, which will actually limit the formation, or stop the progression of arthritis.

You will see in the 'Lift Weights' chapter, you just need to go to failure to reap the benefits of resistance training (failure meaning you can't do another repetition no matter how hard you try). For example, do as many push-ups as you can until you can't do another. Increased muscle mass leads to decreased fat mass, leads to decreased blood glucose levels, leads to increased blood flow, leads to decreased risk of things like diabetes, erectile dysfunction, and heart disease… That's a much better picture now, isn't it?

Just start now!

Or, in some other cases, just stop now!

The following table shows how quitting smoking now affects ones' health. Reduced risks refer to cessation in comparison to continued smoking[13]

Time after quitting health benefits:

Minutes	• Heart rate drops
24 hours	• Nicotine levels in the blood drops to zero
Several days	• Carbon monoxide level in the blood drops to the level of someone who does not smoke
1 to 12 months	• Coughing and shortness of breath decrease
1 to 2 years	• Risk of heart attack drops sharply
3 to 6 years	• Added risk of coronary heart disease drops by half
5 to 10 years	• Added risk of cancers of the mouth, throat, and voice box drops by half
10 years	• Added risk of lung cancer drops by half after 10-15 years. Risk of cancers of the bladder, esophagus and kidney decreases
15 years	• Risk of coronary heart disease drops to close to that of someone who does not smoke
20 years	• Risk of cancers of the mouth, throat and voice box drops to that of someone who does not smoke. • Risk of pancreatic cancer drops to that of someone who does not smoke. • Added risk of cervical cancer drops by about half

---

[13] https://www.cdc.gov/tobacco/quit_smoking/how_to_quit/benefits/index.htm

As you can see, the benefits of quitting smoking can happen immediately. You can improve your overall health tremendously, as well as your cardiovascular, respiratory, and reproductive health, not to mention reducing your overall risk of cancer. See chart below provided by the Centers for Disease Control related to smoking cessation.

HEALTH BENEFITS OF QUITTING SMOKING

- **IMPROVES** health and **INCREASES** life expectancy
- **LOWERS** risk of 12 types of cancer
- **LOWERS** risk of cardiovascular diseases
- **LOWERS** risk of chronic obstructive pulmonary disease (COPD)
- **LOWERS** risk of some poor reproductive health outcomes
- **BENEFITS** people who have already been diagnosed with coronary heart disease or COPD
- **BENEFITS** people at any age - even people who have smoked for years or have smoked heavily will benefit from quitting

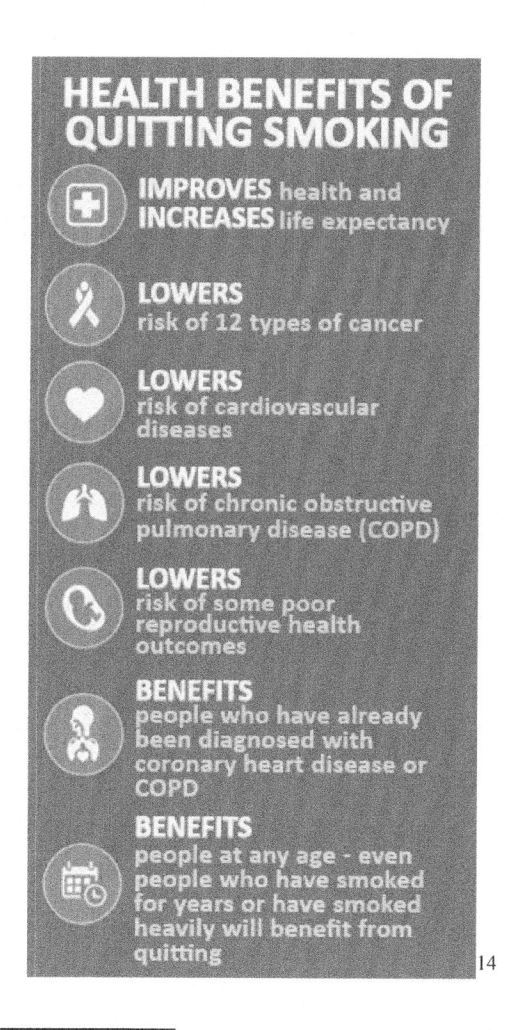

[14]

---

[14] https://www.cdc.gov/tobacco/quit_smoking/how_to_quit/benefits/index.htm

Some of the same things can be said about cutting sugar out of your diet. According to an article found on *Health.com,* removing sugar can lead to reduced risk of diabetes, improved skin, enhanced energy, and decreased belly-fat. [15]

You may be reading this while you're in your early fifties. Guess what? Your late fifties are just around the corner, my friend. Do you want to be another ten pounds heavier, or do you want to be able to walk up and down stairs without dropping to your hands and knees like Chuck Norris just round- house kicked you in the gut? Your choice.

Of course, please remember to run these ideas past your physician and get a physical while you're at it. Eventually, get a physical therapist or strength coach to guide you. For now, find something that gets you moving and get started today.

---

[15] https://www.health.com/nutrition/health-benefits-quitting-sugar

Chapter 6: Inflammation, Sleep, Stress

Inflammation

We live in a high stress world in which most of the time our health isn't at the forefront of our thoughts and actions. Long hours at work, along with poor diet and lack of exercise can lead to many problems that we have discussed. Another very dangerous outcome to this type of lifestyle that we briefly touched on is the role of chronic inflammation.

I'm sure you all are aware of the idea of inflammation, especially after an acute (sudden) injury. Some of you have probably sprained your ankle, or maybe bumped your head and saw a huge lump form or increased swelling at the injury site. This is normal and should be expected. This is your body's way of healing as your immune system floods the area with substances that assist with that process.

The problem with inflammation is when this process is prolonged, and over time, this can be disastrous.

A recent Harvard study has shown 'that chronic inflammation is associated with heart disease, diabetes, cancer, arthritis, and bowel diseases like Crohn's disease and ulcerative colitis.'[16]

---

[16] https://www.health.harvard.edu/staying-healthy/understanding-acute-and-chronic-inflammation .

During a chronic inflammatory state, your immune system is constantly in attack mode, which can result in it starting to assault healthy tissues around an injury site. This can be exacerbated by diabetes and other diseases of poor health, causing more inflammation, which causes more attacks by your immune system, which causes more inflammation, etc.

Some chronic inflammation can be obvious, like bleeding or swollen gums, leading to gingivitis. You may notice this when flossing or brushing. This can lead to the prolonged inflammation that we discussed above which will continue that cycle of immune attack: --> Inflammation --> more immune attack. Unfortunately, not all inflammation is the same. It can be difficult or impossible to see other forms of inflammation without a blood test.

Think about how you feel when dealing with a cold, or flu. Your body is tired and you have little energy. You may have a headache or body aches. This is an effect of your immune system fighting this infection. Your immune system is getting a tremendous workout, so of course you're going to be tired.

What about your day? Are you tired all of the time, or have little energy most days? Are you experiencing indigestion or heart burn, or maybe constipation? Are you noticing you are a bit foggy or confused? This can be the effects of chronic inflammation.

You don't have to have the diseases above to have chronic inflammation. I think we can all see how smoking, or alcohol abuse can cause chronic inflammation with all the toxins being ingested. But did you know that most of the things you eat everyday will do the same?

According to the Cleveland Clinic, here are five common foods that can increase inflammation:

- added sugars
- trans-fats
- red/processed meats
- foods high in Omega-6 (seed oils like sunflower, corn, safflower, peanut, and things like mayonnaise)
- refined carbs like rice, French fries, breads, etc.[17]

Let's breakdown a typical fast-food order: You get a burger (red meat, refined carb bun, mayonnaise) with an order of fries (refined carbs, likely trans-fats and/or Omega-6s due to it being fried in oil) and a large soda (enormous amount of added sugars and other chemicals) along with the condiments.

We could say the same for pizza (meat toppings, refined carbs crust), or the breakfast bagel and O.J. (refined carbs, copious amounts of added sugar) or the steak dinner with potatoes and beer.

---

[17] https://health.clevelandclinic.org/5-foods-that-can-cause-inflammation/

Don't get me wrong, I will and do eat pretty much all of those things, but in deliberate moderation. Pizza is one of my favorite foods, but I don't eat it every day. I will crush an In-N-Out double-double along with some fries, maybe every few months. I'll have a few drinks here and there on the weekends, or a glass of wine with my steak, but I try to be smart about it and not go overboard. Have some fun, but be smart and informed about what it can be doing to your body.

Sleep

A study published in *Science Daily* showed that 'Loss of sleep, even for a few short hours during the night, can prompt one's immune system to turn against healthy tissue and organs.[18] Another study published in *Biological Psychiatry* demonstrated that poor sleep can increase CRP and IL-6 (C-reactive protein and interleukin-6 which are bio-markers for systemic inflammation).[19]

How many of you feel you get a good night sleep every night, or prioritize sleep at all? Maybe some of you watch TV in bed until late, with lights on, after eating a few slices of pizza and drinking a beer less than an hour before trying to fall asleep, only to toss and turn for an

---

[18] Elsevier. "Loss Of Sleep, Even For A Single Night, Increases Inflammation In The Body." ScienceDaily. www.sciencedaily.com/releases/2008/09/080902075211.htm (accessed April 8, 2019).

[19] Irwin MR, Olmstead R, Carroll JE. Sleep Disturbance, Sleep Duration, and Inflammation: A Systematic Review and Meta-Analysis of Cohort Studies and Experimental Sleep Deprivation. Biol Psychiatry. 2015;80(1):40–52. doi:10.1016/j.biopsych.2015.05.014

hour before turning to your phone to check your email. This results in your body being bombarded by blue-light, which will turn off your body's natural ability to produce melatonin (a sleep hormone) along with your digestive system being turned on to work on that pizza you just gobbled not to mention the beer your liver's trying to deal with. All of this leads to degraded sleep and recurring inflammation.

There is a slew of sleep trackers out on the market that can measure your quality of sleep. Some are wearable devices, others are built into the mattress you sleep on. I can tell you from experience that the difference in my sleep quality after just one alcoholic drink is astonishing. If I also had food before bed, the quality plummets even more.

Do yourself a favor and work on your 'sleep hygiene.' Examples of this could be:

- Finding a wind-down routine that works for you: maybe yoga, breathing, stretching or reading a book.
- Turn your TV off, or better yet, no TV while in your bed.
- Increasing your daily activity level will lead to increased fatigue, which will assist with sleep.
- Some people have replaced their lightbulbs with red-light bulbs that emit no blue light.
- Studies have shown that sleeping in a room that's 68 degrees is optimal for restful sleep. Find what works for you and start getting the rest you need and deserve.

- Try not to eat anything at least two hours prior to going to sleep (even better if you can do three-four hours before). And of course, try to avoid alcohol as much as possible.

Personally, I've stopped eating around 4 pm, and I typically go to bed around 9 pm. I know this is not a normal pattern for most of us. I understand that eating dinner as a family may be a priority for some, leading to a later dinner time. For others, their schedules may not allow for closing their 'eating window' that early (more on eating windows later). See what works for you based on your daily commitments, keeping in mind that what is *optimal* for your body may require making some changes.

The following table demonstrates the symptoms of sleep based on the total hours one is able to achieve. As you can see, there is a sweet spot that seems to work best between the 6-10-hour ranges, and that more isn't always better.

Sleep Timeline[20]

No sleep	• Memory lapses, Microsleeps
1-2 hours	• Cognitive errors, confusion, fatigue
3-4 hours	• Insulin resistance, obesity
<5 hours	• Increased risk of mortality
5-6 hours	• Less fat loss/more muscle loss
<6 hours	• Increased hunger and cravings,
	• Weaker immune system
	• Increased BDNF and Fibromyalgia
6-7 hours	• **Optimal cognitive recovery**
7-8 hours	• **Stable blood sugar and recovery**
8-9 hours	• **Optimal muscle growth**
10 hours	• **Enhanced recovery**
11-12 hours	• Fatigue, depression
13+ hours	• Increased risk of disease

---

[20] Courtesy @drjamesdnic

Stress

In a study done by Liu, et.al published in *Frontiers in Human Neuroscience*, it was found that "Chronic stress [can] lead to various diseases such as atherosclerosis, non-alcoholic fatty liver disease (NAFLD) and depression." [21] All of which result in chronic inflammation.

In a study published in the journal *Autoimmunity Reviews*, the authors found that stress has been implicated as a precursor to autoimmune diseases, as up to eighty percent of patients reported "an uncommon emotional stress before disease onset."[22] Further, the study goes on to find that the onset of the autoimmune disease itself causes more stress, which leads to exacerbation of the disease.

An autoimmune disease is one which your own immune system attacks your body. This can lead to devastating diseases such as Multiple Sclerosis (M.S.) Rheumatoid Arthritis (R.A.) and Lupus, to name a few.

Think about your day. Maybe you start by pounding some coffee since you didn't sleep well, before jumping in your car and commuting to work. The stress level has already been turned up. Once you get to work, you go straight to your work station and sit at your computer for

---

[21] https://www.ncbi.nlm.nih.gov/pmc/articles/PMC5476783/

[22] Stojanovich L, Marisavljevich D. Stress as a trigger of autoimmune disease. *Autoimmun Rev.* 2008;7(3):209-213. doi:10.1016/j.autrev.2007.11.007

another few hours before you get up and eat a burger, or a donut, or something else that is quick and easy for lunch along with another cup or two of coffee. You keep grinding at work for another few hours then back to your car for the commute home. Then, like a few paragraphs above, your night routine leads to further stress on your body. You can see how this will lead to less-than-optimal health.

To clarify, some stress is actually good for you. When you put yourself in some situations, like lifting weights at the gym or a run, you're adding stress. This type of stress is good and results in reduced stress when you are done. We've all felt that relief or relaxation when we have completed a difficult workout, for instance.

Additionally, your blood pressure will rise when you are exercising, but it will fall to healthy levels when you are not exercising, reducing your risk of all kinds of diseases. Also, your heart rate will rise during a stressful workout, but will fall to healthy levels for long periods of time afterward.

Bear with me here: If you are running a marathon, your heart rate may be really high for many hours. Let's say 120 bpm for four hours. Doing the math, that's 28,800 beats during that marathon. Now, due to your body being trained enough to complete a marathon in four hours, your resting heart rate will likely be on the lower side. We'll say 60 bpm (normal heart rate 60-100 bpm). If you are at 60 bpm for the rest of the day, your heart will have beaten a total of 100,800 beats (120 bpm x 4 hours) + (60 bpm x 20 hrs.).

Now, if you are at an 'average' heart rate of say 72 bpm as an untrained person, your total beats in a day will be 103,680 (72 x 24 hrs.). That's more than the person who ran that marathon and you did nothing. Extrapolate that over the course of a year, and you would've saved yourself over 1 million beats, or ten days of heart beats if your heart is well trained... and that's if you ran a marathon every day, which I'll assume you did not.

You can now see how a well-trained heart can theoretically buy you time, which in my opinion, is the most valuable of all assets. Physiologically speaking, your heart becomes more efficient and is able to pump more blood per beat, resulting in the need to beat less while delivering the same amount of blood per minute.

That is a prime example of what good stress can do for you.

Now you may be thinking, If I'm stressed out because of work, my heart rate will be up for eight hours, and then go back to resting for the night, which will result in a stronger heart. Sorry. It doesn't work that way. When you exercise, your body adapts by adjusting your blood pressure to supply working muscles. Your arteries and veins adjust by becoming more flexible, and hormones are released that prepare your body for exercise, then bring things back to where they're supposed to be afterwards. Not so with the bad stress. Remember, our bodies were made to move. It will adjust to these good stressors appropriately because that's what it was meant to do.

There are no shortcuts. Challenge your body and it will reward you accordingly.

To summarize, inflammation can be an insidious result of you being in poor health. It can lead to premature aging (some call it 'inflamm-aging') and a variety of diseases that will shorten your life span, as well as your health span.

Sleep plays an important role in preserving and regenerating your body and mind, leading to the ability to live a functional life for a longer period of time. Who wants to spend all of their retirement savings on medications and/or hospital stays? Did you know that the leading cause of bankruptcy in the U.S. is medical costs?[23] Do yourself a favor and work on implementing good sleep hygiene to achieve the quality sleep your body needs daily.

Lastly, stress is a killer that will lead you down a disease-ridden pathway to an early demise. Take time to work on yourself during the day by breathing, exercising, and eating properly. These things can help to reduce the two previous issues of inflammation along with lack of sleep, which can lead to that *optimal* quality of life you are striving for.

---

[23] https://www.cnbc.com/id/100840148

Chapter 7: Metabolic Dysfunction

A problem that has been increasing over the past few decades and is wreaking havoc on our health, and healthcare system is metabolic dysfunction. We are probably all familiar with diabetes and some of the issues that come with it (more on that below). But did you know that 88 percent of Americans are deemed metabolically unhealthy? Let me say that again. According to a study by the University of North Carolina published in the journal *Metabolic Syndrome and Related Disorders* "Data revealed that only 12.2 percent of American adults are metabolically healthy, which means that only 27.3 million adults are meeting recommended targets for cardiovascular risk factors management."[24] Or stated differently, that would be like saying only the areas of greater Los Angeles and Chicago are metabolically healthy, and the rest of the 220 million people in the U.S. are not.

Recommended targets:

- A waist circumference below 40 inches (men) and 34.6 (women)
- Fasting blood sugar below 100
- Blood pressure at or below 120/80
- Triglycerides less than 150
- HDL ('good') cholesterol >40 (men) >50 (women).

---

[24] Prevalence of Optimal Metabolic Health in American Adults: National Health and Nutrition Examination Survey 2009-2016.
https://www.unc.edu/posts/2018/11/28/only-12-percent-of-american-adults-are-metabolically-healthy-carolina-study-finds/

In a recent published report by the American Diabetes Association (ADA), diabetes related costs were found to be $327 billion dollars per year in 2018. And that's up from $245 billion just five years prior in 2012. Further, the study states that one in every seven dollars spent on healthcare in the U.S. is spent on diabetic related costs. [25]

Unfortunately, the news doesn't get much better. According to the CDC, in 2020 "88 million people 18 years or older have prediabetes (34% of the adult US population).."[26] Of those, 25 percent will develop type 2 diabetes.[27] The numbers just keep going up.

So, what can we do?

To be clear, this isn't a book that is going to preach to you about a new fad diet. I'm not going to berate you for not being keto, or try to woo you into joining the paleo tribe. My goal is to arm you with information so you can decide on your own what works for you.

I think we all know what doesn't work. You already know the McDonalds burger and fries that you devour at 8 pm on a Wednesday after a long day at work is bad, as are the fried Oreos that you get from the county fair. Those are easy to discern from what should be eaten.

---

[25] https://www.diabetes.org/resources/statistics/cost-diabetes
[26] https://www.cdc.gov/diabetes/data/statistics-report/index.html .
[27] https://www.health.harvard.edu/blog/many-miss-pre-diabetes-wake-up-call-201303266023

Obviously, one way to help combat this epidemic is to limit caloric intake. Intuitively, I think we all know that 'calories in vs. calories out' is what leads to an increase or decrease in weight (i.e. If the calories you take in are greater than the calories you burn, you will store them and gain weight, and vice-versa). However, another benefit to limiting calories is not just losing weight. It has been found to also promote longevity.

Recently, there has been a tremendous amount of research completed showing a link between limiting overall calories and longevity. I know I just said I'm not pushing a fad diet. The difference is the amount of research that is being done regarding this. When I say research, I mean peer-reviewed studies, not some website guru trying to sell you something.

Truth be told, these studies are difficult to complete due to the fact that there are so many factors that would need to be controlled, not to mention the long timeframe that is needed to show irrefutable evidence. What has been shown, however, has been promising.

In a study completed and funded by the NIA (National Institute on Aging) a calorie restricted diet has presented findings that have shown a loss in weight during the study, as well as weight that was kept off after a two-year follow up. Additionally, the study also stated that this type of diet "reduced risk factors (lower blood pressure and lower cholesterol) for age-related diseases such as diabetes, heart disease, and stroke."[28]

It is well known that weight loss and exercise can reverse type 2 diabetes in people who have been diagnosed. Most of these studies have shown an increase in insulin sensitivity, resulting in a decreased risk of type 2 diabetes, as stated above.

I can't begin to tell you how important this is. Type 2 diabetes is an absolute assassin. This disease, which is completely preventable, can be devastating for almost all systems of your body. It can lead to all kinds of health issues from blindness, kidney failure, amputations and erectile dysfunction to name a few. I've watched as some of my patients have undergone multiple amputations, starting with a toe, then foot, then ending with both legs, due to decreased blood flow from diabetic issues. I've had more patients than I can count who are required to go to dialysis three times per week for the rest of their lives due to kidney failure from diabetes.

I want to emphasize that glucose is used as an energy source, and is the preferred source of energy for your brain. In and of itself, glucose is not a bad thing. It is indeed a necessary molecule for life. Normally, your body produces insulin to deal with glucose (blood sugar) that naturally occurs when you eat certain types of foods (typically, carbs and sugars). Insulin carries this glucose into your cells where it is used and stored for energy. Think of insulin as the key to unlock the cell so glucose can

---

[28] https://www.nia.nih.gov/health/calorie-restriction-and-fasting-diets-what-do-we-know).

enter. Without it, glucose gets stuck in the bloodstream. Here's where the trouble starts.

With type 2 diabetes, your cells become more and more desensitized to insulin (the key doesn't unlock the door) leading to an increase in glucose streaming through your body instead of being stored in your cells. Glucose is kind of like tiny little razor blades that hitch rides on your red blood cells. This can be deadly to small vessels in your kidneys, eyes, penis, and extremities.

I don't think it's a coincidence that erectile dysfunction (ED) is concurrently on the rise. According to the Cleveland clinic, "approximately 40% of men are affected at age 40 and nearly 70% of men are affected at age 70."[29]

Further, diabetic retinopathy is one of the many issues that diabetics have to deal with. Most of us will have age-related vision loss starting typically in our forties. Would I be going out on a limb to suggest that both of these could be a warning sign of poor metabolic health? Maybe you can discuss these issues with your MD for a screening for metabolic dysfunction, instead of just taking a blue pill, or making an appointment with an optometrist for new glasses?

---

[29]https://www.clevelandclinicmeded.com/medicalpubs/diseasemanagement/endocrinology/erectile-dysfunction/

Another issue that is suspected to be involved with metabolic issues has to do with your liver, called nonalcoholic fatty liver disease (NAFLD) and nonalcoholic steatohepatitis (NASH). In a study published in the Greek medical journal *Hippokratia* by authors Paschos and Paleta, it was stated that while "the data are mainly epidemiological, the pathogenesis of NAFLD and metabolic syndrome seems to have common pathophysiological mechanisms, with focus on insulin resistance as a key factor."[30]

Nonalcoholic steatohepatitis (NASH) is a condition that is typically preceded by nonalcoholic fatty liver disease, or NAFLD. The etiology of these two conditions usually starts with excess fatty deposits in the liver (NAFLD - usually diet related) with no other significant signs or symptoms other than occasional pain from an enlarged liver.

NASH, on the other hand can be a serious condition that shouldn't be ignored. There is significant inflammation at the liver, as well as liver damage. As a matter of fact, according to the NIH, "NASH may lead to cirrhosis, in which the liver is scarred and permanently damaged. Cirrhosis can lead to liver cancer."[31]

A major risk factor for these two conditions is obesity. As we have learned, 40 percent of Americans are obese, which would explain why a

---

[30] Paschos P, Paletas K. Non alcoholic fatty liver disease and metabolic syndrome. Hippokratia. 2009 Jan;13(1):9-19. PMID: 19240815; PMCID: PMC2633261.

[31] https://www.niddk.nih.gov/health-information/liver-disease/nafld-nash/definition-facts

study published by Juanola, et al. demonstrated "The prevalence of NAFLD evolves in parallel with obesity."[32]

Keeping with the major organs, acute pancreatitis (AP) is another condition that has been associated with metabolic dysfunction. Gastroenterologists from the Boston Medical Center found in a study that "Metabolic syndrome and its components were associated with AP occurrence."[33] AP manifests in a few different ways, including back pain, abdominal pain, and a swollen abdomen to name a few. It can be extremely uncomfortable and very painful.

Let's look into some more ways to fight metabolic syndrome. Remember, this is something that is completely avoidable and reversible. Here are a few more actionable techniques to help prevent or reverse it.

Most of us know that if we eat less, we will lose weight, or at least not gain much more weight. What I really want you to realize here is that there are a few ways to go about this that seem to work better than the thousands of diets you have heard about that work for a bit, but the

---

[32] Juanola O, Martínez-López S, Francés R, Gómez-Hurtado I. Non-Alcoholic Fatty Liver Disease: Metabolic, Genetic, Epigenetic and Environmental Risk Factors. *Int J Environ Res Public Health*. 2021;18(10):5227. Published 2021 May 14. doi:10.3390/ijerph18105227

[33] Shen Z, Wang X, Zhen Z, Wang Y, Sun P. Metabolic syndrome components and acute pancreatitis: a case-control study in China. BMC Gastroenterol. 2021 Jan 6;21(1):17. doi: 10.1186/s12876-020-01579-3. PMID: 33407178; PMCID: PMC7789414.

person ends up gaining everything back. Being hungry all the time is not conducive to long-term compliance.

For instance, an alternative to a calorie restricted diet, can be a timed-eating diet, or an intermittent fasting diet. Again, I'm not talking here about the latest craze. These are some thoroughly studied eating strategies that have shown promise with overall health and longevity. An example of time-restricted eating can be fasting for sixteen hours, then eating in an eight-hour window (known as a 16:8). This could mean you simply stop eating at 6 pm and resume again at 10 am the next day. These windows can be tweaked to include more or less of an eating window depending on your results/goals. Studies do suggest, however, that the timing of these windows do matter.

In a study by Sutton, et.al., a group that ate between 7am and 3pm "had dramatically lower insulin levels and significantly improved insulin sensitivity, as well as significantly lower blood pressure' versus those who ate in a twelve-hour window between 7am and 7pm."[34]

Dr. Rhonda Patrick further backed up this claim on her website stating:

"For each 10% increase in the proportion of calories consumed after 5pm was associated with a 3% increase in the inflammatory biomarker CRP (c-reactive protein). For each 3-hour increase in night-time fasting duration was linked to a 20% lower odds of elevated glycated

---

[34] https://www.health.harvard.edu/blog/intermittent-fasting-surprising-update-2018062914156

hemoglobin (HbA1C). Studies have shown that consuming food earlier in the day and only during an 11-hour window, can decrease breast cancer risk and recurrence by as much as 36%. Together, these data suggest that time-restricted eating is a viable option to lower biomarkers of inflammation and insulin resistance and lower breast cancer risk and recurrence."[35]

Another study by Dr. Satchin Panda, PhD found that insulin sensitivity is lower around the first two hours after awakening (due to melatonin).[36] This would suggest that eating your first meal at least two hours or more after waking would be better for glucose metabolism, as the effects of melatonin have worn off. Further, it was found that consistency with your fasting/eating windows will allow your body to adapt accordingly so as to optimize the results. That's not to say if your window is altered by an hour or two on the weekends, all is lost. It is to say, however, that for *optimal* results, keeping the same windows is best practice.

Personally, I've been working on skipping breakfast and eating around lunchtime. This has been difficult for me, as breakfast is my favorite meal. I also generally give myself a break on the weekends and I mix in a twenty-four hour fast at least two days out of the month. While this may not be optimal for all, it works for me and I'm satisfied with the results. I've found that starting with a 12:2 (i.e. fasting for twelve hours,

---

[35] https://s3.us-east-2.amazonaws.com/foundmyfitness.public-assets/SAMPLE.Report.pdf

[36] https://www.foundmyfitness.com/episodes/satchin-panda

and not eating until two hours after waking up, then stopping eating at least two hours before bedtime) and adding an hour every week or so to the fast was a great way for me to transition toward a 16:8. I know I said earlier that being hungry all of the time is not conducive to long term compliance, but remember, hunger is just a feeling. People have fasted for over a month and lived to talk about it. Just because you're feeling hungry after eight hours of fasting, doesn't mean its game-over if you don't eat. See what works best for you and stick to it. The pangs of hunger start to decrease. It really does get easier.

For me, weight loss is not a goal I'm trying to reach. At my age I'm trying to keep as much muscle mass as possible, which takes the right amount and type of calories. I am, however, absolutely trying to decrease my diabetes risk, as it runs in my family. Therefore, I need to be careful and deliberate about what I eat so I don't lose weight, and not eat unhealthy food that will put me at risk.

Fasting in and of itself has proven to be a powerful weapon for reducing or reversing disease risk, including some autoimmune diseases like multiple sclerosis (MS). One particularly interesting study by Choi, et al. has shown that a prolonged fast of three days where mice were severely restricted of calories using a fasting mimicking diet (or FMD) found "the FMD reduced clinical severity in all mice and completely reversed symptoms in 20% of animals."[37]

---

[37] https://pubmed.ncbi.nlm.nih.gov/27239035/.

Moreover, the study showed actual remylenation of nerves that had been demylenated from MS. Myelin is an insulator that surrounds a nerve, increasing its conduction speed. MS is a disease that destroys myelin, reducing nerve conduction speed resulting in physical debility.

Of course, this particular study was done on mice, so further studies are being done to find the effects on human subjects. This could be a game-changer for a lot of people and hits very close to home for me personally. My wife has MS and I had a cousin who died from complications of MS.

Other proven benefits from fasting range from increased fat burning, increased human growth hormone (HGH), reduced systemic inflammation and increased autophagy (ah-TAH-fa-gee).

Autophagy is the act of your body deleting dead or underperforming cells (called senescent cells), which results in them being replaced by healthy cells that execute as needed. This is another very important benefit. Cells that aren't doing their job properly slow the whole system as you could imagine how an old set of spark plugs would decrease the power of a car. A poorly performing cell does the same to your body. Replace those plugs (or cells) and voila! Everything's at peak, or *optimal* performance. For an extensive hour-by-hour list of what's going on during a fast, see the graph below

So there you have it. We've discussed how metabolic syndrome can affect pretty much all of your major organs pathologically. From heart disease, strokes (brain), NASH (liver), diabetes (kidneys), and pancreatitis, along with your penis and eyes to boot. You can see how this wholly avoidable and reversible syndrome can utterly destroy your body. I wasn't bringing these things to your attention to scare you, but hopefully it made an impact enough to where you can make the necessary changes to your lifestyle and diet to avoid the pitfalls associated with metabolic syndrome.

As you have read, there are a few different actionable things you can start today that will have an immediate impact, as well as help point you in the right direction for the rest of your life. Longevity through various eating strategies is an exciting field that is making progress quickly. By limiting your risk factors for diseases of poor health, both your lifespan and health span can be extended, along with your ability to optimize your functional ability. Remember, no one wants to spend all of their retirement income on medications.

Note: please consult with your MD or a registered dietician to confirm that these strategies are safe for you, as certain conditions or situations may necessitate a specific type of diet not conducive with the aforementioned strategies

Here's a breakdown of what your body does each hour of fasting (times based from last calorie intake):

Four-eight hours

Blood sugars fall

- All food has left the stomach.
- Insulin is no longer produced.

Twelve hours

- Food consumed has been burned.
- Digestive system goes to sleep.
- Body begins healing process.
- Human Growth Hormone begins to increase.
- Glucagon is relaxed to balance blood sugars.

Fourteen hours

- Body has converted to using stored fat as energy.
- Human Growth Hormone starts to increase dramatically.

Sixteen hours

- Body starts to ramp up the fat burning.

Eighteen hours

- Human Growth Hormone starts to skyrocket.

Twenty-four hours

- Autophagy begins.
- Drains all glycogen stores.
- Ketones are released into the blood stream.

Thirty-six hours

- Autophagy 300 percent increase.

Forty-eight hours

- Autophagy increases 30 percent more.
- Immune system reset and regeneration.

- Increased reduction in inflammation response.

Seventy-two hours

- Autophagy maxes out.[38]

---

[38] [38]https://www.inhousestudiofitness.com.au/blog/2019/5/15/the-hour-by-hour-benefits-of-intermittent-fasting

Chapter 8: Lift Weights

<u>Disclaimer</u>: I know this chapter will be hotly contested. There are a few different ways to make an exercise routine that will work for you. I am recommending thoroughly studied programs that have been shown to work based on data collected in controlled environments. I'm sure there are other studies that can be identified and cited for their effectiveness at achieving muscle growth, just as there will be the gym crowd who will cite their own personal program that they've been using for years at the gym for muscle growth. If you have been doing something that works for you, please continue. What I am presenting will save you some time and hopefully be the safest and most efficient way to achieve results.

***

I'll bet at some point in your life you went to the gym and just started lifting a dumbbell or two with no real plan in place, other than to throw some weight around. You probably lasted a few sessions before you got really sore, or worse, got injured and had to quit. Or maybe life got busy and you started putting it off and the next thing you know, you're paying for a gym membership that you haven't used in years. Sound familiar?

As stated in the 'Be an Athlete of Life' chapter, muscle wasting happens to us all, typically starting at around thirty, thanks to a natural decrease in testosterone. To compound this problem, at that age, some of us may be starting to raise a family, or putting in ridiculous hours at the office trying to climb the corporate ladder (or likely doing both of these things). This can lead to lack of sleep and increased stress, both of which can be disastrous to the body's system.

We've all been in situations where we've had a deadline, or a busy time at work or home. You can feel your heart racing, your body is exhausted, you're short-tempered with family, friends, co-workers, etc. You're feeling the effects of cortisol. Cortisol, the stress hormone, is an antagonist to testosterone. Typically, they are inversely proportional. (Note: testosterone is not just for men. Women also produce and benefit from testosterone, just as men produce and benefit from estrogen. Both of these are important hormones that help with optimizing both men's and women's health).

During sleep, more precisely deep and REM sleep, our bodies produce human growth hormone (HGH). You may think you are getting sleep, but are you really getting the type of sleep you need? Like I said before, there are a lot of really cool devices out now that can measure how much, and the type of sleep you are getting. It can be eye-opening to see how little things can make a huge difference in our sleep quality.

Going back to our real-life example: Hectic commute, stressful job, family commitments, poor diet, lack of exercise, and deprived sleep. Cortisol is dominating your life.

Bottom line: increased cortisol leads to decreased testosterone, which leads to lack of quality sleep (i.e. decreased HGH), which will eventually lead to an unhealthy body. Is this you? Remember when you were twenty-three and you told your friend, 'if I ever look like that, slap me...' Consider this your slap.

To offset this, lift heavy weights.

To increase testosterone, build muscle, and maintain strength you have to do resistance training. I'm sure you may know this, but are you doing it properly? I'll bet you're not. This is where a physical therapist, CSCS or an educated personal trainer comes in handy (of course, be sure your doctor is aware and on board with this).

New studies have shown that a good way to build muscle is to lift to failure, lifting until you can't do another repetition. Going to the gym and pushing the same weight around every day is better than nothing, and can maintain what you have, but won't truly build more muscle (*hypertrophy*). Now, this doesn't mean you have to try to lift your maximum weight every session either. There's more than one way to skin a cat.

Going to failure can be doing a one rep max, lifting the maximum amount of weight you can complete for one repetition, OR it can mean doing a much lighter weight for more reps until you can't do another rep no matter how hard you try. You can throw a few pounds on the barbell and bench press until you can't press anymore (with a spotter of course), or you can drop down and do push-ups until you collapse. Both of these will accomplish the same thing, although the push-ups will incorporate a lot more muscle groups.

Doing compound type exercises (deadlifts, squats, cleans, kettlebell swings) are typically the best type for increasing testosterone. Many studies have shown that these, and other resistance exercises offset muscle atrophy and increase testosterone levels which can result in increased muscle hypertrophy, not to mention increased sex drive, increased bone mass, and better sleep. The increased sleep leads to increased HGH levels, which in turn benefits your body by keeping your muscles, tendons and ligaments strong and injury free. This allows you enough energy and strength to get back in the gym to do it over and over. See how it all works together? Repeat this cycle enough and you can feel as good as you did in your twenties.

Although we may have to make a few modifications due to the increased wear-and-tear on our older bodies, you absolutely can feel and even look as good as you did when younger by doing things properly and consistently.

To be fair, studies have shown that there is an array of tweaks that can be done to optimize gaining strength versus gaining muscle (hypertrophy) as well as gaining speed/power versus endurance. Those can be researched at a greater level as you become more consistent with your workout regimen and what you wish to accomplish becomes more defined. Until then, starting a program as mentioned above can be a great way to build a foundation.

Also, I understand that everyone has an opinion about what is the best way to go about this, especially the folks who spend hours in the gym. They may tell you that everything I've told you is wrong, and you should do what they are doing. Don't fall into this trap! It is a very quick way of getting injured in most cases. While some of what they are telling you may be correct, I've worked with many a patient who has listened to them only to end up hurt and discouraged. This is where a good strength coach (CSCS), or educated personal trainer can really help. When I say educated, I don't mean internet trained. I mean one that has a good understanding of kinesiology (human movement) as well as physiology. Anyone can push someone until they can't move for a week, but it takes an experienced trainer/coach to guide you properly and safely toward your goals.

Like I said before, Father Time is undefeated. Eventually there comes a point where you're not going to look like you did in your twenties, or in your fifties. Your body will eventually produce less and less testosterone and HGH naturally no matter what we do. I don't care. It's my goal to go as long as I can and be as functional as possible. Do you want to be the seventy-year-old who can't walk with his grandkid, or do you want to be the seventy-year-old who picks up a bag of concrete for some fifty-year-old guy who can't?

Chapter 9: Limit Meds

Another benefit of being healthy is not needing a multitude of expensive medications. I don't know about you, but I don't want to spend my hard-earned retirement savings on a cluster of medications that all have a side-effect of some sort. I can't tell you how many patients I've had that will actually forgo buying a needed medication due to their inability to afford it. Unfortunately, some medications may be a necessity, and in no way am I telling you to stop taking your prescribed medications. However, you may be able to limit your need for some, or all medications, by living a healthy lifestyle.

The progress we have made over the past few centuries in medicine has been miraculous, no doubt. Even so, I think that a lot of medications are over-prescribed and can lead to long-term issues. It's always an eye-opener to me how many medications some of my patients are taking. It's amazing that they are actually hungry after taking so many. That's unfortunately what too many MDs do, just prescribe medicine.

For example, the prescription of proton pump inhibitors for heartburn or gastro-esophogeal reflux disease (GERD) has been shown to disrupt the gut microbiome so badly that it can lead to devastating infections like *Clostridium difficile*, (think horrible diarrhea that you can't get rid of without very strong antibiotics).[39] The use of these strong antibiotics leads to a further devastation to the gut biome which can lead to many

---

[39] https://pubmed.ncbi.nlm.nih.gov/26657899/

other issues, not to mention a build-up of resistance to these antibiotics. What would cause you to need these meds for GERD? Well, another highly prescribed medication like ibuprofen, which has listed as side-effects "upper gastrointestinal hemorrhage, upper gastrointestinal tract ulcer" among many other things.[40] So in this case, you may need to take one of these meds to treat the side effects of the other? Raise your hand if you've ever been prescribed ibuprofen by your MD? It was prescribed almost 25 million times in 2019.[41]

Please understand, I'm not saying that by taking ibuprofen you will develop GERD, but I am trying to illustrate a point that some meds are given to treat the side effects of others. There is a very good chance that a change in lifestyle, including exercise and a healthy diet, can eliminate the need for both of these.

Were you prescribed ibuprofen because your shoulder hurt? Go see a physical therapist and fix the shoulder. This goes along with the saying 'treat the issue, not the symptoms.' In my humble opinion, it's time that we change healthcare from just waiting to treat the sickness, to focusing on not getting sick in the first place. That is, to focus more on *wellness* and less on *sickness.* Some countries do a great job of this. Others, like the Unites States, leave much to be desired.

---

[40] https://www.drugs.com/sfx/ibuprofen-side-effects.html
[41] https://www.healthgrades.com/right-care/patient-advocate/the-top-50-drugs-prescribed-in-the-united-states

Look no further than the COVID-19 pandemic as an example of this. Surely this virus is deadly, and in no way am I downplaying the seriousness of it. I saw firsthand the damage that this virus caused, and even lost a family member to it. However, if you look at how healthy people reacted to being infected versus those with pre-existing conditions, the data speaks for itself.

For instance, obesity was shown to be devastating when partnered with COVID-19. According to the CDC, it tripled one's risk of hospitalization, and furthermore, the risk of hospitalization and/or death was greater in those obese patients *under* 65.[42] Seeing as how 40 percent of Americans are obese and 75 percent are overweight, it's no wonder this virus is so deadly.

Please know that I am not being insensitive toward those poor folks who lost their lives to this nasty virus, some of who were perfectly healthy. Just know that I am trying to make a point that a little work toward a healthier lifestyle can help protect us from these fatal outbreaks.

A bit more perspective from AARP regarding medications:

"The average annual retail cost of drug therapy for a prescription drug in 2017 was almost $20,000 per year. Paying for one prescription drug completely out of pocket would cost more than the average person's

---

[42] https://www.cdc.gov/obesity/data/obesity-and-covid-19.html.

yearly Social Security retirement benefit that year, $16,848. It would also cost more than three-quarters of the annual median income for Medicare beneficiaries of $26,200."[43]

Hopefully, you have, or will have good insurance that will cover most of this. But the costs of the out of pocket/co-pay can still be upwards of $1000 for some meds. Now what if you have to take nine or ten different medications? You see how this can all add up and eat away at your income? I see patients every day that are on a fixed income of social security only. It can be a sad existence. After they have their wages garnished by the low-income apartment they are living in, they barely have enough left over for anything else, leading to the alarming choice of eating, or buying their meds. Either way, the choice will have harmful consequences.

Not to beat a dead horse but using those numbers above can help further clarify my point. If you have a shoulder issue and you go see a physical therapist, the cost to your insurance will likely be somewhere between $100 and $150 per session. Typically, it will take up to twelve visits (or less) to treat and correct the injury, as well as to educate the patient on ways to avoid repeating the injury. All in all, the total cost will be somewhere between $1200 and $2000. Now if you take a medication, it may end up costing insurance and/or you up to $20k if you use AARPs reference. I know it may not exactly be comparing apples to apples, but if you took ibuprofen that led to a stomach issue,

---

[43] https://www.aarp.org/politics-society/advocacy/info-2019/jenkins-soaring-drug-prices.html

which lead to a prescription medication to treat that issue... you see where I'm going. People in the United States worry that social security will not be around for much longer. I'm more concerned that Medicare over spending and mismanagement will break us if we don't get healthier as a society.

This is no plea for socialized healthcare. In a study conducted by The Commonwealth Fund, which is an organization that promotes quality healthcare to the most vulnerable people of the world, Canada ranked near last in most major categories. Canada, the poster child for socialized healthcare in North America, was found to be "especially abhorrent in making their health care safe, timely, or efficient."[44]

So how can we avoid having to spend chunks of money on costly medications? It can be as easy as getting up and going for a short walk and progressing little by little every day. If you have type 2 diabetes, ask your healthcare provider for resources that can point you in the right direction for diet and exercise that may be able to allow you to reduce, or get off certain medications completely. Think of what you can do with all of that extra cash.

---

[44] https://www.medicaldaily.com/5-major-countries-worst-health-care-395258

Chapter 10: Stretch

I took my first yoga class in my early thirties. It was an eye opener to say the least. Not only did I realize how unbelievably stiff I was, but it was extremely challenging from a strength perspective.

I was like a lot of guys in my twenties and thirties. I hit the weights hard and was physically active. However, when I was done with these activities, I never embraced the importance of stretching. Taking stretching and flexibility seriously is one thing I would absolutely tell my younger self to do if I could.

As a physical therapist, I can't tell you how many people, from all age groups, ask me how they can address a back issue that they've been dealing with for years.

According to a study published in *The Lancet,* "low back pain is the single leading cause of disability worldwide."[45]

Another common complaint I hear are shoulder problems. Surely all of the heavy bench press guys like me did in their twenties contributed to this, sometimes right away, other times later in life. Other things could just be the fact that people are sitting for prolonged periods of time

---

[45] http://www.thelancet.com/themed/global-burden-of-disease

with horrible posture, leading to poor alignment up and down their body.

Think about this and tell me if it sounds familiar: You get in your car and drive to work while hunched over your steering wheel for your thirty-minute commute (give or take). You head up to your desk (having taken the elevator instead of the stairs) and sit there hunched over your keyboard for eight hours plus. You take the elevator back down to your car and sit in traffic for another thirty minutes hunched over your steering wheel only to get home and plop on the couch and watch TV until 10pm.

The number of things wrong with this picture is staggering. I'll break it down:

First, hunched over your steering wheel while sitting in traffic is not only terrible on your shoulders (think rounded shoulders due to tight chest) but on your back as well (think tight hips and hamstrings). Add to that a bit of stress from your commute, and you have all the trappings of an orthopedic issue ready to explode. But wait! There's more.

Next, you get to your desk and sit in the same dreadful position over your computer for eight hours, likely with a bit more stress sprinkled in. You probably have your arms extended while sitting and working that keyboard, which will increase stress on your neck and shoulder area, as well as enhance the tightness in your shoulders, hips, and hamstrings.

Once that's done, back to the car we go for another round of stop-n-go all the way home, hands strangling the steering wheel, hunched posture, spewing curses at the person who just cut you off. Finally, you get home and what do you do? You sit in front of the TV in the same poor posture you've been in all day. Is it any wonder why your back is a mess and your shoulders and neck are tighter than your grandparents at Christmas?

Of course, there can be many other reasons why one's back or shoulders are affected. But, for the most part, these issues can be addressed and avoided altogether with some simple stretching and strengthening strategies.

Focus on your large muscle groups and start with those. Think chest, latissimus (back muscles that start at your low back and end under your armpits) hamstrings, quads, hips/glutes, calf muscles. A skilled physical therapist, chiropractor, or an educated personal trainer can help guide you with this. Also, yoga, Pilates, or barre may be good options, as long as you are physically able to participate in such activities. Find what works for you.

Remember, if it's something you like to do, it will make it a whole lot easier. Recruit a friend, coworker, or your spouse/significant other to join you and help hold you accountable.

Did I mention why I became a physical therapist? Well, I also had a pretty severe back issue in my twenties caused by repetitive motion from pulling orders while working in a warehouse. I was laid up a few different times and had mild to moderate back pain almost daily. I visited a back surgeon who looked at my x-rays and MRI and said I would need surgery to fix the issue. No, thank you.

I did some research and figured out strategies to help alleviate the back issue, through stretching and strengthening. Continued interest in this subject (and others) lead me to pursue a kinesiology degree to be an athletic trainer, and eventually to grad school and post-graduate school to become a doctor of physical therapy. This not only allowed me to help myself, but others as well, and I could make a living while doing so.

Poor flexibility also leads to poor balance, which can lead to falls. As one gets older, this can be devastating, leading to broken bones. A very common issue is a broken hip from falling. A study published by the NIH concluded that this can lead to a 3-fold mortality rate.[46] Typically, one becomes fearful of falling after this, which leads to one being more sedentary, which leads to poor circulation and the onset of many other health issues. This eventually leads to the quickened mortality rate.

Stretching is one of the single best things you can do to help avoid musculoskeletal issues, no matter your age or lifestyle. You may be like the people described above, your issues may be stemming from a

---

[46] https://www.ncbi.nlm.nih.gov/pmc/articles/PMC3118151/

stressful life, or from lifting weights or being physically active. Either way, stretching is an essential activity that should be done to decrease tightness and poor posture, which can help lead to more beneficial movement patterns and reduce injury risk. Even better, being more flexible will make you stronger, faster, less susceptible to injury and a better all-around athlete of life.

Chapter 11: Go Outside

According to an article in *Time* magazine "By 2050, 66% of the world's population is projected to live in cities."[47] Further, a study by the EPA showed that the average American spends 93 percent of their time indoors. The need for protected outdoor spaces is a necessity to allow a reconnection, or at least a distraction from a life spent mostly indoors disconnected from the way we lived for so many years in the past.

I can tell you that I absolutely feel better when I'm outdoors rather than cooped up in my house. I'm fortunate enough to be able to walk on a sandy beach most days, as well as over the ground barefoot when I'm walking out to go surfing.

Recently, there has been a trend suggesting that connecting to the earth, what some call 'earthing' has beneficial and therapeutic effects. This is based on the physical science of 'grounding' one's self, similar to that of a grounding wire in an electrical circuit.

The body is made up of electrically charged molecules, as is the earth and its magnetic field. By standing barefoot on the ground, you help to realign these systems.

---

[47] https://time.com/5259602/japanese-forest-bathing/

I know this sounds a little like some hocus-pocus hippie nonsense, but there have been studies that back up this claim. A study published by the National Institutes of Health (NIH) Chevalier, et.al. found that "Grounding increases the surface charge on RBCs [red blood cells] and thereby reduces blood viscosity and clumping. Grounding appears to be one of the simplest and yet most profound interventions for helping reduce cardiovascular risk and cardiovascular events"[48] Another study showed that even being submerged in the water can have the same benefits as being on the ground.[49] So go for a swim in the ocean, lake, or another body of water and you can further benefit from this effect.

Another way to get some of these effects is what has been referred to as 'forest bathing.'. According to National Geographic, the term was coined in the 1980s by the Japanese as a way to avoid tech-burnout and get people to get out and not only appreciate the forest, but to reconnect and protect it.[50] These studies have also demonstrated an improvement in psychological well-being, decreased inflammation, decreased stress, and reduced pain.

Surely the fact that you can't be 'connected' (i.e. on your phone) while swimming in a lake or ocean helps with this. If you are out hiking or hanging out in the forest, leave your phone in your car and try to focus all five senses on nature around you. Learn to appreciate the silence,

---

[48] https://pubmed.ncbi.nlm.nih.gov/22757749/
[49] https://www.healthline.com/health/grounding#types
[50] https://www.nationalgeographic.com/travel/article/forest-bathing-nature-walk-health

which for most of us will be a complete 180 from what we are used to in our daily lives.

Chapter 12: Hydration

According to the National Institutes of Health, most Americans are chronically dehydrated. As a matter of fact, their studies have suggested that up to seventy-five percent of Americans are exactly that.[51] The reasons for this vary from people thinking coffee or soda will suffice, to people just not feeling thirsty. Some other reasons can be medical issues as the following suggests:

- failure to replace water loss due to altered mentation, immobility, impaired thirst mechanism, drug overdose leading to coma
- excess water loss from the skin: heat, exercise, burns, severe skin diseases
- excess water loss from the kidney: medications such as diuretics, acute and chronic renal disease, post-obstructive diuresis, salt-wasting tubular disease, Addison disease, hypoaldosteronism, hyperglycemia
- excess water loss from the GI tract: vomiting, diarrhea, laxatives, gastric suctioning, fistulas
- intraabdominal losses: pancreatitis, new ascites, peritonitis
- excess insensible loss: sepsis, medications, hyperthyroidism, asthma, chronic obstructive pulmonary disease (COPD), drugs[52]

Another reason can be even simpler: breathing. When we exhale, we lose water through our lungs. You can get a good visual of this during a

---

[51] https://www.ncbi.nlm.nih.gov/books/NBK555956/
[52] https://www.ncbi.nlm.nih.gov/books/NBK555956/

cold day, but it happens during any type of weather. Think of how many breaths we take daily. The average breaths-per-minute is about sixteen in a normal adult. Extrapolate that times twenty-four hours and you're looking at over 23,000 breaths in which we will lose a small amount of water. If you compound this with any type of exercise (excessive sweating/breathing) or reasons above, you can see how this can add up quickly to a lot of water. The human body is made up of up to 65 percent water, and it is important to maintain this volume for optimal function.

Water's many essential jobs include:

- oxygen delivery
- saliva/mucous production
- joint lubrication
- spinal cord and brain protection
- body temperature regulation
- maintaining healthy skin
- regulating blood pressure
- GI regulation (reduces constipation and ulcer risk)
- performance enhancement during exercise
- proper kidney function
- allows certain minerals and nutrients to be more bio-available.

The effects of dehydration can be numerous, ranging from a headache to heart palpitations, with most common symptoms of dehydration being:

- fatigue
- thirst
- dry skin and lips
- dark urine or decreased urine output
- headaches
- muscle cramps
- lightheadedness
- dizziness
- syncope (fainting)
- orthostatic hypotension, and palpitations.
- vital signs may show hypotension (low blood pressure), tachycardia (fast heart rate), fever, and tachypnea (fast breathing).

There are a few simple ways to tell if you are dehydrated. It can be pretty easy to see based on the color of your urine. If your urine is dark-colored, go drink some water. Your urine should be fairly clear most of the time. Some foods, medications or vitamin supplements can affect the color of your urine, so keep this in mind if you feel as if you have been drinking enough water.

Personally, I can tell if I'm dehydrated when I start feeling a headache coming on. Instead of reaching for the aspirin or Tylenol, I reach for a big glass of water and drink it. Headache gone in less than five minutes.

I also make it a point to try to finish at least four liters of water daily, more if I've exercised intensely. While some of the time I don't feel thirsty, I'll drink a liter at a time just because. As you will see in the 'bio-hacks' chapter, the first thing I do when I get out of bed is down a liter of water before I start my day. This not only ensures I get a leg up on my hydration, but it helps get the metabolism fired up for the day, starting my circadian clock. Remember, you just slept for six to eight hours and likely hadn't had a drink during that time.

It has also been shown by numerous studies, that most of us don't need anything more than water for proper hydration. There is an abundance of energy drinks and sports drinks that are mostly loaded with sugar, calories and caffeine that can be deleterious to your health and hydration. While an electrolyte drink can be beneficial in certain circumstances (like running a marathon, for instance) water is almost always a safer and a better choice. According to Patrick Skerrett, former executive editor for *Harvard Health*, sports drinks can have up to ten tablespoons of sugar and up to 150 calories.[53] Further, Tim Noakes, professor of exercise and sports science at University of Cape Town South Africa, was quoted as saying if most people drank water and avoided sports drinks "they would get thinner and run faster." [54]

Staying hydrated can help your kidneys stay healthy and can help you avoid things like kidney stones. I don't know about you but getting a kidney stone terrifies me. I've never had one, thankfully, and hope to

---

[53] https://www.health.harvard.edu/blog/trade-sports-drinks-for-water-201207305079
[54] https://www.health.harvard.edu/blog/trade-sports-drinks-for-water-201207305079

keep it that way. In a study published in the *Annals of Internal Medicine,* findings showed that "increasing fluid intake to enable 2 liters of urination a day could decrease the risk of stone recurrence by at least half with no side effects."[55] That should be motivation enough to stay hydrated.

Water plays a vital role in our daily lives. Without it, most humans will typically die within three days. As we age, we can lose our ability to detect thirst. Further, some of the medications that people take can act as a diuretic, meaning it can speed up your body's ability to get rid of water, leaving you more dehydrated. Other things, like drinking alcohol or coffee can have this same effect. Make it a habit to drink many times throughout the day and not just drinking when you are feeling thirsty. This in turn will help you maintain optimal function so you can attack the day, accomplish your goals and feel great while doing it.

---

[55] https://www.acpjournals.org/doi/10.7326/M13-2908

Chapter 13: Alcohol

In no way is this a chapter based on judgement or hypocrisy. I want to get that out of the way immediately. As I have stated previously, I enjoy a drink or two occasionally. Remember, my goal is to arm you with as much information as possible to allow you to make informed decisions regarding your health.

There are studies that have been published which support the consumption of a drink per day of red wine as a cardio-protectant.[56] These studies, however, are demonstrating how certain substances within the red wine are beneficial. These substances can also be found in many other food or supplement sources, which don't include the alcohol, which of course is a hepatotoxic (toxic to your liver). Certain antioxidant compounds called polyphenols and resveratrol can be found in red wine. They can also be found in abundance in foods like blueberries, elderberries, cocoa, flaxseed, certain nuts, as well as green tea to name a few. These antioxidants are extremely important for helping to reduce cell damage caused by aging, as well as helping to lower blood pressure, inflammation, and insulin resistance. Remember, a proper diet or supplementation program will get you these things, without the damage that the alcohol itself can inflict.

---

[56] https://www.mayoclinic.org/diseases-conditions/heart-disease/in-depth/red-wine/art-20048281

Speaking of damage, I think we have all seen the extreme end of the spectrum of what excessive alcohol abuse can do. Liver dysfunction, cirrhosis, cancers, pancreas/heart issues, cognitive decline, social problems etc. But what about the more subtle damage it can do which can lead to other serious issues?

In a study published by Dr. Judith S. Gavaler, PhD, moderate alcohol consumption was found to have an *estrogenic* effect (it increased estrogen production) on subjects. [57] In fact, Dr. James Woods from the University of Rochester Medical Center showed that increased estrogen results in fat distribution along the female patterns of breasts, buttocks, thighs and stomach.[58] I've heard the term 'beer-belly' actually referred to as 'estrogen-belly' due to alcohol's effect on increased estrogen. This is nothing against estrogen, as it is a hormone that we all produce, both male and female. But the overproduction of one and underproduction of another is where problems will occur.

More studies have shown that moderate and heavy/chronic alcohol consumption reduces testosterone production.[59] This, in turn, can lead to decreased sperm motility, infertility, erectile dysfunction, and the other diseases mentioned above. Heavy drinking is defined as more than fifteen drinks per week for men and more than eight for women. Moderate was defined as no more than one per day for women and two

---

[57] https://pubs.niaaa.nih.gov/publications/arh22-3/220.pdf
[58] https://www.urmc.rochester.edu/ob-gyn/ur-medicine-menopause-and-womens-health/menopause-blog/may-2015/what-does-estrogen-have-to-do-with-belly-fat.aspx
[59] https://www.ncbi.nlm.nih.gov/pmc/articles/PMC6571549/

per day for men. It goes without saying that if you are making more estrogen and less testosterone, your hormones are out of whack and your health will suffer.

I know there will be critics out there who will try to dispel all of these arguments. Let me help you. One particular study conversely found that low doses of alcohol actually increased testosterone in men.[60] I won't argue with the data.

What I will say is alcohol is toxic and your body views it as a poison. Your liver's number one goal once alcohol hits the system is to rid your body of it ASAP. Like most things, if we are smart and practice moderation, alcohol can be something that we can enjoy. I've mentioned before that I enjoy a glass of a bold red wine with a rib-eye steak. I will also occasionally throw back a bourbon with friends and neighbors on the weekend. Watching a baseball game with a beer and hot dog is hard to beat. These things I appreciate, however I do my best to practice moderation. I figure I work too hard on my fitness to undo everything by drinking too much. There are times I overdo it, and boy, do I pay the next day. Sorry, I don't have any proven tricks to make hangovers as mild as they were in our twenties.

---

[60] https://pubmed.ncbi.nlm.nih.gov/12711931/

Chapter 14: Added Sugar

Avoid it. The end ...

But seriously, our bodies depend on glucose to survive, and glucose is indeed a type of sugar molecule, but added sugar should be moderated or avoided as much as possible. There is literally no need for added sugar in our diet for our survival.

The FDA states "added sugars include sugars that are added during the processing of foods (such as sucrose or dextrose), foods packaged as sweeteners (such as table sugar), sugars from syrups and honey, and sugars from concentrated fruit or vegetable juices. They do not include naturally occurring sugars that are found in milk, fruits, and vegetables. The Daily Value for added sugars is 50 grams per day based on a 2,000 calorie daily diet."[61]

There have been studies that have suggested that sugar can be as addicting as some drugs and many others have proven the link between excess sugar consumption and many types of diseases like heart disease,[62] and a strong correlation with obesity.

---

[61] https://www.fda.gov/food/new-nutrition-facts-label/added-sugars-new-nutrition-facts-label
[62] https://www.hopkinsmedicine.org/health/wellness-and-prevention/finding-the-hidden-sugar-in-the-foods-you-eat

While it has been difficult to prove unequivocally that sugar can be "addictive" in the same way that cocaine or alcohol can be, it has been shown that sugar consumption has been tied to the release of dopamine the same way addictive drugs like cocaine or opioids do.[63] The same study showed that sugar consumption can lead to bingeing behavior, craving, sensitization, and withdrawal symptoms. All of these are classic characteristics of addiction.

Of course, the food companies know this and exploit these effects of sugar on us. We all willfully know that if we eat a candy bar, we are ingesting sugar. However, in a more sinister act, food companies will hide sugar within foods to elicit the same response. This will lead us to unknowingly crave or overeat this food due to the chemical release created by it.

These added sugars hide in plain sight in numerous foods you eat and you likely don't even realize it. For instance, go to your cabinet and take a look at some of the things in there. Typical foods like cereals, ketchup, sodas, milk, and even foods you may think are healthy like yogurt can be loaded with added sugars. They can come in the form of high fructose corn syrup, brown sugar, molasses, and brown rice syrup to name a few. I encourage you to do a search for the different names of added sugars, then be on the lookout for those on your food labels. The paragraph below from Johns Hopkins Medicine gives some examples:

---

[63] https://www.ncbi.nlm.nih.gov/pmc/articles/PMC2235907/

To identify added sugars, look at the ingredients list. Some major clues that an ingredient is an added sugar include:

- it has syrup (examples: corn syrup, rice syrup)
- the word ends in "ose" (examples: fructose, sucrose, maltose, dextrose)
- 'sugar' is in the name (examples: raw sugar, cane sugar, brown sugar, confectionary sugar).

Other examples of added sugar include fruit nectars, concentrates of juices, honey, agave and molasses.[64]

The American Heart Association has recommended no more than nine teaspoons (38 grams) of added sugar per day for men, and six teaspoons (25 grams) per day for women.[65] You may think that's a lot of sugar and it may be hard to get that amount, but if you have a bowl of 'heart healthy' Honey Nut Cheerios with milk, you're at 15 grams of added sugar already. And that's just breakfast. Drink a Coke, and you can add 43 grams of added sugar from that one 12 oz can to your daily count. If you can make one change today, stop drinking soda.

---

[64] https://www.hopkinsmedicine.org/health/wellness-and-prevention/finding-the-hidden-sugar-in-the-foods-you-eat
[65] https://www.ahajournals.org/doi/pdf/10.1161/circulationaha.109.192627

I want to clarify the difference in sugars so as to avoid any confusion. There are many sugars that occur naturally in foods. Fruits have sugar in them, and our body breaks down carbohydrates into sugar. While your body doesn't really know the difference between added and naturally occurring sugar, or carbohydrates and the sugar from fruit at a molecular level, there is indeed a big difference.

Let's say you get hungry and want to reach for a snack. You open your refrigerator and pantry to see what you can grab quickly and easily. In the fridge you find some delicious strawberries, and in the pantry, you find a conveniently packaged strawberry multi-grain bar. One cup of those strawberries contains 8 g of naturally occurring sugar, along with 160 percent of your daily RDA of vitamin C, 2 g of fiber and a bit of calcium and iron to boot; all with a grand total of 50 calories. Now take that strawberry multi-grain bar. It is so tremendously overprocessed, that there are no less than forty-three ingredients listed on the box, with sugars named seven different times.[66] While it has 12 g of added sugar, it too offers some protein, vitamins and 1 g of fiber. All that leads to almost triple the calories at 130 per bar.

The same can be said for oranges and orange juice. If you eat an orange, you will get 12 grams of sugar, but you will also get 3 g of fiber, over 1g of protein, as well as more than one day's-worth of vitamin C. If you drink 12 ounces of orange juice, you will get double the calories (112 vs

---

[66] https://www.nutrigrain.com/en_US/products/soft-baked-breakfast-bars/kellogg-s-nutri-grain-cereal-bars-strawberry-product.html?utm_source=bing&utm_medium=search&utm_campaign=NG%7CBing%7CSearch%7CSnack%7CNonBrand%7CUS%7CFlavors%7CBMM

62 in an orange), one-sixth the amount of fiber and almost double the amount of sugar. It would be very difficult to eat as many oranges as it takes to get enough juice to fill a 12 oz glass, since it takes about four oranges for one cup of juice. Therefore, you would need to eat about six oranges to equal the same amount of juice in a 12 oz glass of OJ. Probably not going to happen.

Obviously, it's much easier to drink a glass or two of OJ than it is to eat twelve oranges. From a nutritional standpoint, the two glasses of OJ are loaded with sugar and empty calories and are a poor choice for your body.

These examples illustrate a few of the biggest differences between highly processed foods with added sugars, and foods with naturally occurring sugars. The calorie count is typically much higher, the food is much more processed into something unnatural that is difficult for your body to recognize, and the ingredient list is full of things that are not typically found in unprocessed foods. Not to mention the hidden sugars that will cause your body to crave more of these processed disasters. It's almost always a better choice to go with the natural foods.

According to Registered Dietician Adda Bjarnadottir, MS, RDN, 'There's no reason to avoid the sugar that's naturally present in whole foods. Fruit, vegetables, and dairy products naturally contain small amounts of sugar but also fiber, vitamins, minerals, and other beneficial compounds. The negative health effects of high sugar consumption are due to the massive amount of added sugar that's present in the Western diet. The most effective way to reduce your sugar intake is to eat mostly whole and minimally processed foods."[67] Eating 'real' food as opposed to what can be called 'Franken-foods', or heavily processed items that barely resemble food, is going to be the better choice.

You hopefully know by now the dangers of type 2 diabetes and how increased sugar intake can lead to insulin resistance, metabolic dysfunction and obesity. Sugar as a direct cause to type 2 diabetes has been difficult to implicate, but we do know there is a strong correlation between obesity and increased sugar consumption. We also know that the obesity rate in the U.S. is 40 percent, and up to 75 percent are overweight as we read in 'Sitting is the New Smoking' chapter.

Additionally, 34.2 million Americans have type 2 diabetes (about one in ten) and 88 million have pre-diabetes (one in three) according to the CDC.[68] To put a bow on all of these statistics, in a study by Faruque, et.al, it was found that "The US population consumes more than 300% of [the] daily recommended amount of added sugar."[69]

It's not that hard for me to see the correlation between metabolic diseases and increased sugar consumption when you study the data. There can be, and surely there are a multitude of confounding factors that can muddy the waters. This is why nailing down a specific and

---

[67] https://www.healthline.com/nutrition/56-different-names-for-sugar#Glucose-or-fructose-Does-it-matter?
[68] https://www.cdc.gov/diabetes/library/features/diabetes-stat-report.html
[69] https://www.ncbi.nlm.nih.gov/pmc/articles/PMC6959843/

inarguable study implicating sugar intake and diabetes can be difficult, as the controls for such a study are challenging.

Anecdotally, I can tell you that I've never been as lean and felt as good as when I cut out added sugar and excess carbs for a period of time. I have done my best to continue this diet, but like many of the other things we've talked about, I indulge at times. Put a pizza in front of me, and look out. I occasionally enjoy a slice of cake, or a chocolate chip cookie (or four). This has been very challenging for me, as my sweet tooth is legendary, and my wife is a baking queen. I try to make smarter choices, have decreased my overall carbohydrate intake and have done my best to eschew the excess sugar.

Further, I have used a continuous glucose monitor (CGM) to observe how my body reacts to certain foods. This is a wearable device that stays on your body allowing a glucose reading through a smartphone app at any given time. This has allowed me to see how certain foods affect my glucose levels, allowing me to make smarter choices as to what I can eat, and what I should avoid in order to steer clear of metabolic issues.

Personally, I have researched all of the information that I need to make my choice. I encourage you to do some research and draw your own conclusions, whether that be through reading studies, or cutting out excess sugars from your diet and gauging the results.

Chapter 15: BPAs, PFAs, Plastics and Other Forever Chemicals

We are surrounded by plastics daily, from our cars to our Tupperware. Plastics literally changed the way we live and allowed us to be more efficient, make things stronger and more lightweight, and allowed us to progress in the medical field with new and innovative devices that prolonged life.

Unfortunately, there are also many downsides to living with all of these plastics.

I'm sure many of us are familiar with the tragedy of our oceans and rivers being littered with plastics, and the damage this causes. Still, many people continue to buy and use single-use plastics daily, contributing to this environmental epidemic. You may have seen the images of fish belly's full of micro-plastics, or the turtle with a plastic straw stuck in its nose.

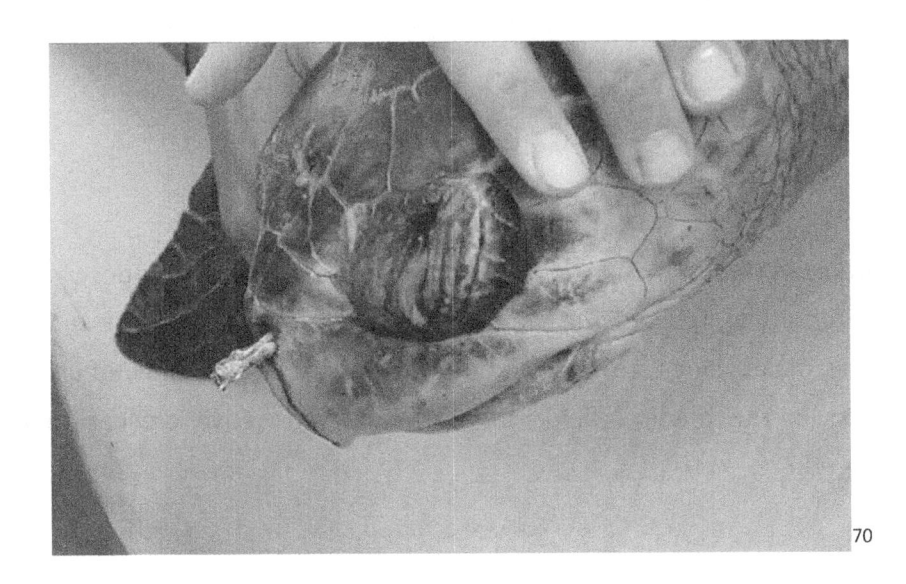

Sea turtle with a plastic straw in its nose

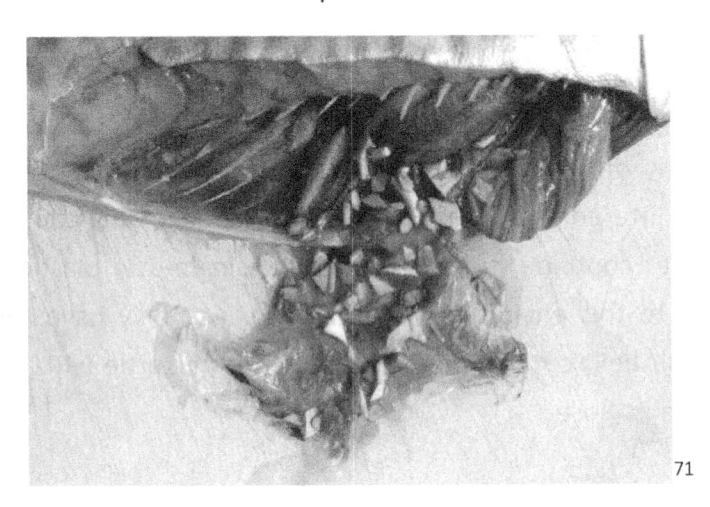

Fish belly full of micro-plastics

---

[70] https://sciencevibe.com/2015/08/17/no-to-straws-marine-biologists-pull-a-12-centimeter-straw-out-of-a-turtles-nose/

[71] https://www.cbsnews.com/news/microplastics-arctic-circle-ocean-pollution-plastic-waste-around-the-world/

While these images are disturbing, they don't show what these same plastics and other chemicals are doing to human bodies.

Phthalates

Phthalates are a type of acid that are added to plastics to increase their flexibility and durability. They are also added to other things that we use daily, like packaging, medical devices, lotions, soaps, and shampoos, to name a few. Recently, they have been the suspected cause of many health issues. Unfortunately, they are very hard to avoid due to the fact that they are in things that we use or are around daily, and are even be in the air we breathe (see following table).

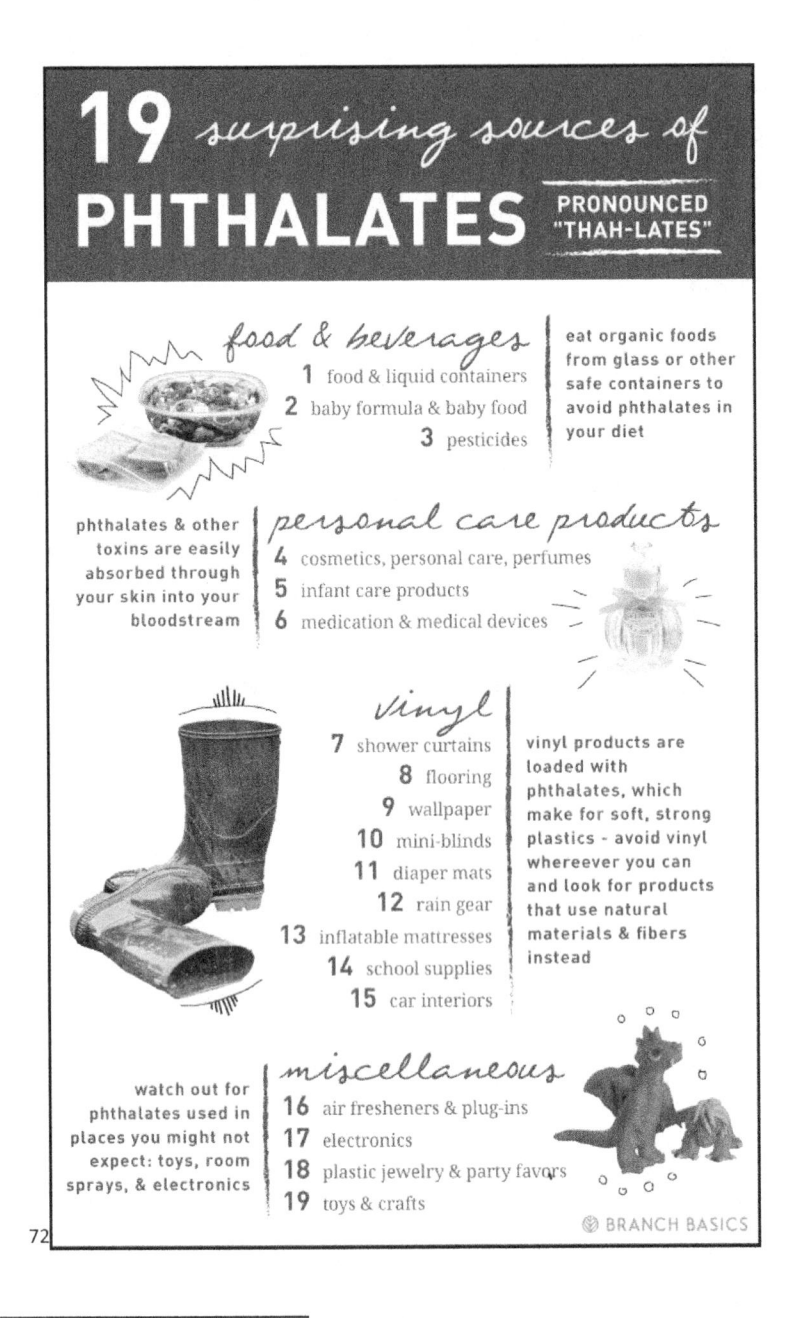

19 *surprising sources of* PHTHALATES
PRONOUNCED "THAH-LATES"

food & beverages
1. food & liquid containers
2. baby formula & baby food
3. pesticides

eat organic foods from glass or other safe containers to avoid phthalates in your diet

personal care products
4. cosmetics, personal care, perfumes
5. infant care products
6. medication & medical devices

phthalates & other toxins are easily absorbed through your skin into your bloodstream

vinyl
7. shower curtains
8. flooring
9. wallpaper
10. mini-blinds
11. diaper mats
12. rain gear
13. inflatable mattresses
14. school supplies
15. car interiors

vinyl products are loaded with phthalates, which make for soft, strong plastics - avoid vinyl whereever you can and look for products that use natural materials & fibers instead

miscellaneous
16. air fresheners & plug-ins
17. electronics
18. plastic jewelry & party favors
19. toys & crafts

watch out for phthalates used in places you might not expect: toys, room sprays, & electronics

© BRANCH BASICS

---

[72] https://branchbasics.com/blogs/home/common-household-chemicals-phthalates-19-surprising-sources

[73] Shanna Swan, PhD, with Stacey Colino. Scribner, February 2021

Dr. Shanna Swan has written an incredible book titled *Count Down: How Our Modern World Is Threatening Sperm Counts, Altering Male and Female Reproductive Development, and Imperiling the Future of the Human Race.*[73] In this book, Dr. Swan documents how men today have half of the testosterone levels that their grandfathers did. She also shows how these chemicals are affecting male testosterone levels such that, if the current trend continues, can lead to a zero level of testosterone in the next two decades. She used exquisite research techniques to come up with proof of deformities related to exposure to these substances. She did a tremendous amount of heavy lifting for this book, and rather than just spew out quote after quote, I encourage you to read it and see for yourself how harmful these chemicals can be to our bodies.

Think for a minute if you know anyone who has had trouble conceiving a child in the last few years? In my circle of friends (Gen X), I can say that most of them were able to conceive naturally with a few exceptions. In my wife's circle of friends (Millennial or Gen Y) quite a few of them have had to go the fertility assistance route. As for my kid's friends (Gen Z) it's as if more of them had to go with fertility assistance then didn't. There is a pretty stark difference, albeit anecdotally, in just one or two generations. There are indeed studies that can back this up.

According to a study conducted by the University of New South Wales, Australia, women face the following challenges:

- 12% of women experience difficulties becoming pregnant or carrying a child to term
- 1 in 8 couples in America encounter fertility hurdles

- 12-15% of all couples are unable to conceive after a year of unprotected sex.
- 10% of all couples are unable to conceive after two years of unprotected sex
- 33% of Americans have turned to fertility treatments, or know someone who has.[74]

Further, according to the NIH, men are part of the problem as well:

- 9% of men of reproductive age experience fertility issues
- in approximately 40% percent of infertile couples, the male partner is either the sole cause or a contributing cause of infertility.[75]

Also, the total birth rate has declined from 3.5 births in 1950, to 2.0 in 2007.[76] Of course, there can be a group of factors that contribute to this (i.e. couples deciding to not have children, or to have fewer children in general) but when coupled with the above stats, a sharp decline can likely be expected to continue.

---

[74] Assisted reproductive technology in Australia and New Zealand: cumulative live birth rates as measures of success Georgina M Chambers, Repon C Paul, Katie Harris, Oisin Fitzgerald, Clare V Boothroyd, Luk Rombauts, Michael G Chapman and Louisa JormMed J Aust 2017; 207 (3): 114-118. || doi: 10.5694/mja16.01435 Published online: 24 July 2017

[75] https://www.nichd.nih.gov/health/topics/menshealth/conditioninfo/infertility

[76] https://www.urc-chs.com/sites/default/files/Guatemala_DeclineinHumanFertility_Sept10.pdf

BPA

Some of us may have heard of Bisphenol A (BPA), which is a chemical that is used in plastics. It can be found in things such as water bottles, plastic food containers, food wrappers, and some dental products. According to the Mayo Clinic, BPA has been found to have "possible health effects on the brain and prostate gland of fetuses, infants and children. It can also affect children's behavior. Additional research suggests a possible link between BPA and increased blood pressure, type 2 diabetes and cardiovascular disease."[77]

The problems occur when the things that are being stored in the BPA container are contaminated by these chemicals leaching into them. For instance, a very common way this happens is when we microwave foods in plastic containers (don't ever do this again). Another way is leaving a plastic water bottle in a hot car. This speeds up the leaching of chemicals into the water, then you drink this contaminated water. Also, plastic baby bottles that were produced before 2011 were made with BPA containing materials, which means we all drank out of them, and if you had kids, they probably did too.

---

[77] https://www.mayoclinic.org/healthy-lifestyle/nutrition-and-healthy-eating/expert-answers/bpa/faq-20058331

Now, you may be thinking, *I drank out of them and I'm fine!* As discussed in an earlier chapter about things we did when we were younger; whether you see it or not, your body was affected in some way from these things, be it a decreased level of testosterone, or maybe an increased risk for cancer.

Enough with the scare tactics. There are indeed BPA-free plastics and here are the ways you can tell:

Most plastic bottles are labeled with a recycling number on the bottom. Look for the numbers 1,2, 4 or 5, which are considered BPA-free. Better yet, you can go with paper or glass bottles and ditch plastics altogether.

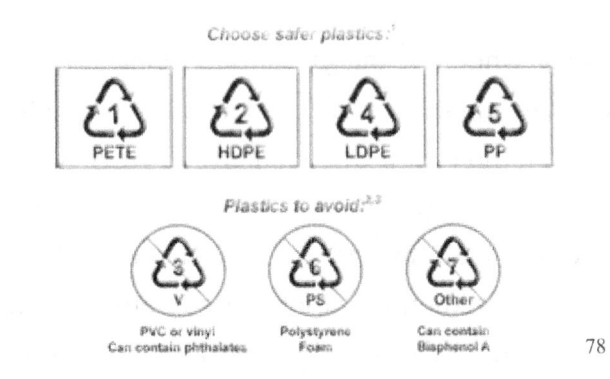

Choose safer plastics:

| 1 PETE | 2 HDPE | 4 LDPE | 5 PP |

Plastics to avoid:

| 3 V | 6 PS | 7 Other |
| PVC or vinyl Can contain phthalates | Polystyrene Foam | Can contain Bisphenol A |

[78]

PFAs

Similar to BPAs, per-and polyfluoroalkyl substances (PFAS) are substances that are added to things we encounter daily, such as

---

[78] https://www.nj.gov/humanservices/opmrdd/images/photo_library/bpafree/PEHSU_recyclingchart300.gif

carpets, cosmetics, our clothes, and non-stick pots and pans to name a few. The CDC has linked these substances to reproductive, liver, thyroid, immune system and kidney disorders.[79]

Further, it has been shown that these substances have been shown to be stable and never degrade. They can accumulate in the body, as well as in water systems and throughout the environment. They have been labeled 'forever chemicals' because of this.

Luckily, legislators have recognized the risk these substances pose and many states are working toward legislation that would limit, or eliminate these substances altogether.[80]

This isn't a book about fertility, and I'm assuming that those of you who are reading this that are in your late forties or older aren't too concerned about the ability to produce more offspring. You should be, however, concerned with the impact these things are having on your hormones that can and will affect your health (and that goes for all of us, not just those of us in our forties or older).

A decrease in testosterone levels will affect our health at any age. A steady stream of poisons from plastics will no doubt wreak havoc on our bodies somehow, whether we see it now or not. Do yourself and the environment a favor and use something other than plastics as much as possible. Your body will thank you for it. Education is key. It is

---

[79] https://www.cdc.gov/biomonitoring/PFAS_FactSheet.html

[80] PFAS Action Act

important to do your homework so you can know what is in the foods and products that you use and are around daily that can affect your health. Be proactive and learn about the products you buy and consume so you can make healthy decisions for you and your family.

Chapter 16: A Typical Day

To prepare yourself for the upcoming day, follow a few simple rules to ensure the best possible start. First, have a jug of water next to your bed so that you can chug it first thing. Make it at least 32 oz or more. While you're asleep, you will get dehydrated. After all, you have been asleep for six to eight hours and haven't had anything to drink. Your body is busy regenerating/recovering and it is using water to help with these processes. You will obviously need to continue hydrating throughout the day, but by drinking that water first thing, you are giving your body the hydration it needs to get off to a great start.

Next, as soon as you can, get outside and go for a brisk walk to expose yourself to light. I know some of you may not be able to do this depending on where you live and the time of year. Maybe you have a treadmill that you can use to at least get the blood flowing and kick start the metabolism. If you can't get the sunlight exposure, try turning on bright lights of any kind. Do this even If you can't do the walk. This is important to keep your body coordinated with the *circadian rhythm* and a proper sleep/wake pattern for optimal function.

For thousands of years, our ancestors went to bed when it got dark, and got up when it got light. They weren't bombarded by blue light emitting screens that they stared at slack-jawed all night. This way of life lasted for centuries, and humans typically thrive when this rhythm is followed.

Oft-cited research from the famous Nurses' Health Study showed that nurses who worked "for more than 15 years on rotating night shifts had a 38% higher risk of dying from heart disease than nurses who only worked during the day."[81]

This helps to demonstrate the role this rhythm continues to play in a healthy lifestyle, even in this modern world.

Continuing on, depending on when you ate last, go ahead and eat breakfast, or skip it and wait until your eating window is open. Coffee is fine, just be wary of what you're putting in it (sugar, whipped cream, caramel, etc.). A sweetener is okay, but try to go with a plant-based sweetener like stevia. Just be sure that it doesn't have dextrose, which has been shown to increase your blood glucose.

Go about your day as usual, but remember to try to stand up at least once per hour. Take a minute or two every hour to take a few deep breaths. Take the stairs as able. I have a few friends who do squats during phone calls and drop to do a few push-ups every few hours as well.

When you get home, try eating dinner as soon as you are able so as to give yourself at least two or three hours between your last meal and bed time. Also, try to go on a walk, or do some other activity after

---

[81] https://www.ajpmonline.org/article/S0749-3797%2814%2900623-0/fulltext

dinner to help burn off the upcoming glucose spike that will occur after your meal.

Remember, metabolic health, in my opinion and according to many studies, is one of the biggest contributors to longevity. That walk/activity will get your muscles contracting, which will burn that glucose for fuel instead of leaving it to flow through your veins or wait to be stored as fat for a later time.

Lastly, look into some blue light blocking glasses that you can wear as the sun goes down. The lights in our house, not to mention all of the screens that we look at, emit blue-light which has been shown to disrupt our circadian rhythm. Feel free to take a melatonin supplement if needed, but know that your body is also producing that wonderful hormone, as long as the blue-light is being restricted.

Limit alcohol consumption before bed as well, as it is a notorious sleep disruptor. My heart rate variability (HRV) score will plummet after just a single drink. HRV is a sign of health that tracks the variations in heartbeat. A higher HRV equates to better health. This can be tracked with wearable devices nowadays. Practice good sleep hygiene and prepare yourself for a good night sleep so you can wake up and be the best version of yourself.

Chapter 17: Bio-Hacks

To increase testosterone: (Please consult your MD to be sure these things are safe for you)

1. Lift weights and exercise
2. Eat a proper diet
3. Sleep
4. Stay away from BPAs, PFAs, pthalates, and other forever chemicals
5. Avoid seed oils (canola, corn, soy, grapeseed, safflower, etc.)
6. Get vitamin D (supplement or sun)
7. Take a zinc supplement
8. Reduce stress
9. Reduce/avoid alcohol
10. Intermittent fasting

To increase sleep:

1. Reduce exposure to blue light in evening and night hours
2. Stop caffeine consumption after noon
3. Reduce stress through meditation or breathing exercises
4. Take a melatonin supplement if needed
5. Avoid alcohol
6. Stop eating at least two to three hours before bed
7. Set temperature to 68 degrees

To improve overall health:

1. Drink a liter (32 Oz's or more) of water FIRST THING IN THE MORNING before you do anything
2. Go on a walk or do another form of exercise in the morning to start your day
3. Ask your doctor about a continuous glucose monitor, or look at buying a blood glucose monitor to see how certain foods affect your glucose levels
4. Get a CBC/lipid panel done at least twice per year
5. Get a colonoscopy
6. Try a carb/calorie limiting diet
7. Try intermittent fasting, or a time-restricted diet
8. Go on a walk or do...
9. Light exercise after dinner (or every meal if possible)
10. Drink two tablespoons of apple cider vinegar daily (a natural anti-inflammatory and wonderful probiotic for gut health)
11. Walk barefoot outdoors
12. Stretch
13. Get a yearly physical
14. Look into a good multivitamin

Conclusion

My goal with writing this book was to share with you the knowledge that I have gained which will allow you to make more educated decisions in the way you live your life. Most of these things I wish someone would have told me years ago. Hopefully, after reading this you have come away with a greater understanding on ways to improve your overall health and functionality.

I invite you to further look into these subjects, as you may find a few ways to personalize your new lifestyle even more. Many of the authors that I have cited go much more in depth on the individual topics that were discussed and have written wonderful pieces that covered these subjects meticulously. If there was a certain chapter that you want to learn more about, I invite you to research that subject and learn more on your own.

Lastly, good luck to you on your journey toward a healthier life. It can be very difficult at times, and there will be slip-ups along the way. Nobody's perfect. The end result, however, will be a much more enjoyable and functional time on this planet, which at the end of the day, is what we are all striving for.

About The Author

Dr. Mathew Barry, DPT, MS, CSCS was born and raised in the San Francisco Bay Area and currently resides in San Diego, California with his beautiful wife, Susan. Mathew has 3 adult children who he is extremely proud of. He currently works as a physical therapist specializing in neurological disorders, as well as treating a variety of other physical issues.

Mathew obtained both a bachelors and master of science degree from Sacramento State University, before going on to obtain a doctoral degree from A.T. Still University, Arizona School of Health Sciences.

One word that best describes Mathew is curious. If he doesn't know the answer to something, he is known to immediately start researching the topic to not only understand it, but be able to educate others. His love of knowledge has best been demonstrated when serving as an Adjunct Professor for a Physical Therapist Assistant program over the past decade.

Mathew has always been active and athletic and is constantly looking for ways to challenge himself physically and mentally. He has completed multiple triathlons, a half-marathon, and participates in various team and individual sports. He's even competed in a body building contest.

Matt currently spends his free time surfing, playing baseball, playing guitar, and practicing mixed-martial arts.

Please follow Mathew on facebook at Mathew Barry, as well as Instagram @drmathewbarry, LinkedIn at Mathew Barry, DPT, MS, C.S.C.S., and twitter @DrMathewBarry1 , for continued information on new bio-hacks, more ways to stay healthy, and tips to increase longevity (YouTube channel coming soon, stay tuned).

Made in the USA
Monee, IL
18 January 2024